Diastasis Recti

The Complete Guide to Recovering From Abdominal Separation and Restoring Your Abdominal Wall

Ethan D. Anderson

Xspurts.com

Created by Xspurts.com

A New Zealand Designed Product

Other Versions Available

Why limit yourself to just one format?

This book is now available in physical, digital, and audiobook options.

Choose the way you love to read and dive into the story today. You won't regret it!

Digital ISBN: 9781776969814
Physical ISBN: 9781776969807
Audio ISBN:

To obtain a different format of this book at a discounted price, please get in touch with us at:

http://isbn.xspurts.com/

Contents

Have Questions / Comments?

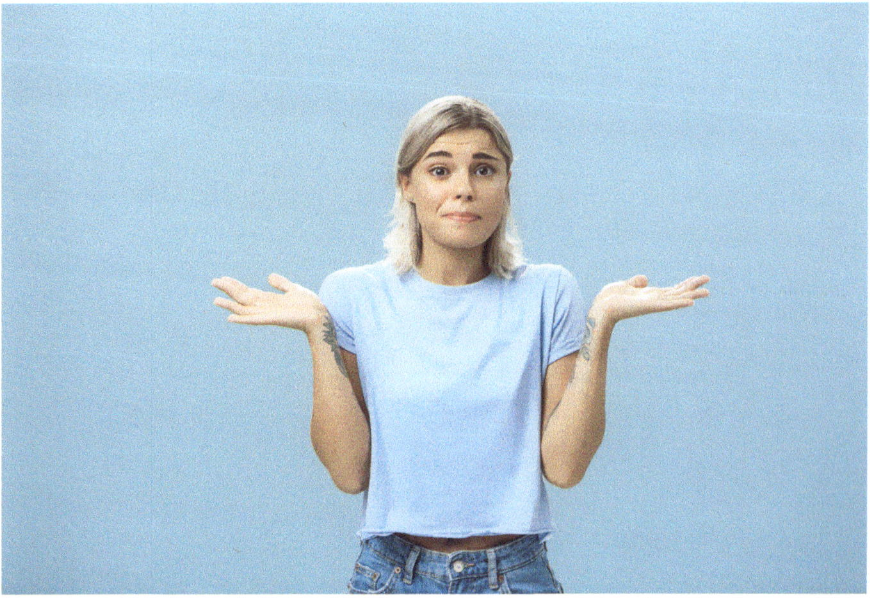

This book was designed to cover as much information as possible, but I know I have probably missed something, or some new amazing discovery has just come out.

If you notice something missing or have a question that I failed to answer, please get in touch and let me know. If I can, I will email you an answer and also update the book so others can also benefit from it.

Thanks For Being Awesome :)

Submit Your Questions / Comments At:

https://questions.xspurts.com

Get Free Stuff

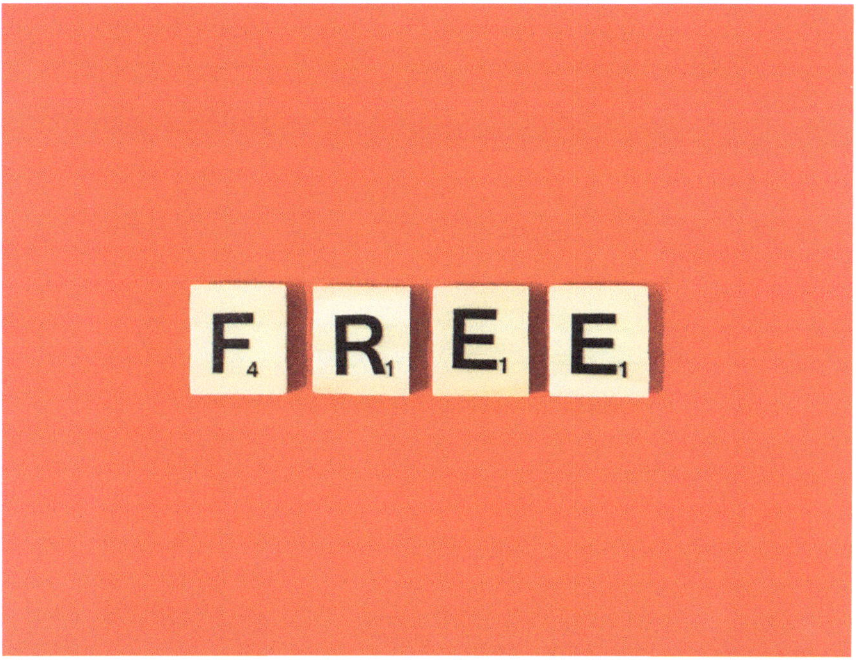

We love writing and have produced a huge number of books.

For being one of our amazing readers, we would love to offer you more books we have created, 100% free.

To claim this limited time special offer, simply go to the site below and enter your name and email address.

You will then receive loads (as we love our readers so much :) of our great books, content and audio direct to your email account, 100% free!

Get Loads of FREE Stuff at:

https://free.xspurts.com

Chapter One

What is Diastasis Recti?

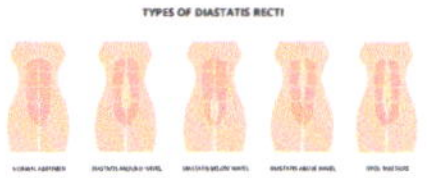

Diastasis recti is a condition that occurs when the two sides of the rectus abdominis muscle, which runs down the center of the stomach, separate. This separation causes a gap in the abdominal muscles, which can lead to a bulge or protrusion in the midsection. This condition is common in women who have given birth, but it can also occur in men and women who have never been pregnant.

The rectus abdominis muscle is responsible for supporting the organs in the abdominal area, as well as providing stability and balance to the body. When this muscle separates, it can cause a number of problems, including weakened abdominal muscles, poor posture, and lower back pain. It can also lead to difficulty with activities such as lifting heavy objects, exercising, and even sitting up in bed.

Diastasis recti is most commonly associated with pregnancy, as the growing uterus can put pressure on the abdominal muscles and cause them to separate. This condition is also more common in women who have had multiple pregnancies, those who have had a large baby, and those who are over the age of 35.

While diastasis recti is often associated with pregnancy, it can also occur in men and women who have never been pregnant. In fact, it is estimated that up to 60% of men may have some degree of diastasis recti. This can occur as a result of poor posture, excess weight in the abdominal area, or repetitive movements that put strain on the abdominal muscles.

Symptoms of diastasis recti can include a visible bulge or protrusion in the midsection, lower back pain, poor posture, and difficulty with activities such as lifting heavy objects or exercising. In some cases, diastasis recti may be accompanied by other conditions, such as pelvic floor dysfunction or urinary incontinence.

Treatment for diastasis recti typically involves exercises and lifestyle changes that help to strengthen the abdominal muscles and improve overall posture. Physical therapy may also be recommended to help with muscle re-education and to prevent further separation of the abdominal muscles.

In some cases, surgery may be recommended to repair the separation of the abdominal muscles. This is typically only done in cases where other treatments have failed, and it is usually only recommended for severe cases of diastasis recti.

Preventing diastasis recti can be difficult, but there are some steps that can be taken to reduce the risk of developing this condition. These include maintaining a healthy weight, practicing good posture, avoiding heavy lifting or repetitive movements that strain the abdominal muscles, and participating in regular exercise that is appropriate for your level of fitness.

In summary, diastasis recti is a common condition that can cause a number of problems, including weakened abdominal muscles, poor posture, and lower back pain. While this condition is most commonly associated with pregnancy, it can also occur in men and women who have never been pregnant. Treatment typically involves exercises and lifestyle changes to strengthen the abdominal muscles and improve posture, but in severe cases, surgery may be necessary.

Chapter Two

Definition and explanation of diastasis recti

Diastasis recti is a condition where the right and left sides of the rectus abdominis muscles, commonly known as the "six-pack muscles", separate from each other. This separation causes the midline connective tissue of the abdominal wall, called the linea alba, to stretch and weaken, resulting in a visible bulge in the belly area.

Diastasis recti is most common in women who have been pregnant, particularly those who have had multiple pregnancies, but it can also affect men and women who have never been pregnant. It is estimated that up to 60% of postpartum women have diastasis recti to some degree.

The condition is often associated with weakened abdominal muscles and can cause lower back pain, constipation, and urinary incontinence. In severe cases, it can also cause hernias or other complications.

Diastasis recti can be diagnosed through a physical examination by a healthcare provider, but it is also possible to check for it at home. To do so, lie on your back with your knees bent and your feet flat on the floor. Place your fingers on your belly, with your fingertips pointing towards your feet. Slowly lift your head and shoulders off the floor, as if performing a crunch. If you feel a gap between your muscles that is wider than two fingers, you may have diastasis recti.

While diastasis recti can be a cosmetic concern for some, it is important to note that it is also a medical condition that can cause discomfort and complications. Treatment options vary depending on the severity of the condition, but they often involve exercises to strengthen the abdominal muscles and support the connective tissue.

In some cases, surgery may be necessary to repair the separation and restore the abdominal muscles to their proper position. However, surgery is usually only recommended for severe cases where the gap is greater than two centimeters and other treatment options have been ineffective.

Prevention of diastasis recti is possible with proper exercise during pregnancy and after childbirth. Exercises that focus on strengthening the transverse abdominis, pelvic floor muscles, and obliques can help to support the abdominal muscles and prevent the separation from occurring or worsening.

In conclusion, diastasis recti is a condition where the rectus abdominis muscles separate from each other, causing a visible bulge in the belly area. While it is most common in women who have been pregnant, it can also affect men and women who have never been pregnant. Treatment options vary depending on the severity of the condition, but they often involve exercises to strengthen the abdominal muscles and support the connective tissue. Prevention is possible with proper exercise during pregnancy and after childbirth. If you suspect you may have diastasis recti, it is important to consult with a healthcare provider to receive a proper diagnosis and determine the best course of treatment.

Chapter Three

How common it is and who is affected

Diastasis recti is a common condition that occurs most frequently in women during and after pregnancy. In fact, up to two-thirds of pregnant women will experience some degree of diastasis recti. However, this condition can also affect men, women who have never been pregnant, and even newborns.

Diastasis recti occurs when the rectus abdominis muscles, which are the "six-pack" muscles that run down the front of the abdomen, separate from each other. Normally, these muscles are held together by a band of connective tissue called the linea alba. However, during pregnancy, the growing uterus can put pressure on the abdominal muscles and cause them to stretch and separate. This can lead to a gap between the muscles, which is known as diastasis recti.

In addition to pregnancy, other factors that can contribute to diastasis recti include weight gain, abdominal surgeries, and chronic coughing or sneezing. Some people may also be more genetically predisposed to developing this condition.

While diastasis recti is most commonly associated with pregnancy, it can also affect men and women who have never been pregnant. In fact, one study found that up to 35% of men had a diastasis recti, although it tends to be less severe in men than in women.

Newborns can also be born with a temporary diastasis recti, which is usually caused by the pressure of being in the womb. However, this usually resolves on its own within a few weeks after birth.

Overall, while diastasis recti is a relatively common condition, it is not always a cause for concern. However, for some people, it can lead to other issues such as back pain or pelvic floor dysfunction, so it is important to be aware of the condition and take steps to manage it if necessary.

Diastasis Recti in Men

Diastasis recti is typically associated with women who have gone through pregnancy, but it can also occur in men. While it is less common in men, it is still a condition that can cause discomfort and affect the function of the abdominal muscles.

Diastasis recti in men can occur due to similar factors as in women, including obesity, improper lifting techniques, and chronic coughing or straining. It can also be a result of certain medical conditions, such as chronic obstructive pulmonary disease (COPD) or cystic fibrosis.

Symptoms of diastasis recti in men may include a protruding belly, lower back pain, and weakened core muscles. Some men may also experience difficulty with digestion and bowel movements, as well as urinary incontinence.

Diagnosis of diastasis recti in men is typically done through a physical exam and imaging tests, such as an ultrasound or CT scan. Treatment options for men with diastasis recti are similar to those for women and may include exercises and physical therapy to strengthen the abdominal muscles.

In some cases, surgery may be necessary to repair the abdominal muscles and improve core function. It is important for men with diastasis recti to work closely with a healthcare professional to develop a treatment plan that is right for their specific needs and goals.

Overall, while diastasis recti is more commonly associated with women, it is a condition that can affect men as well. It is important for both men and women to be aware of the potential risk factors and symptoms of diastasis recti and to seek proper diagnosis and treatment if necessary.

Chapter Four

Causes and risk factors

Diastasis recti is a condition in which the rectus abdominis muscles, which run vertically along the front of the abdomen, separate or move apart from each other. This can result in a bulge or protrusion in the abdominal area, and can be accompanied by symptoms such as lower back pain, constipation, and urinary incontinence.

While diastasis recti can affect anyone, it is more commonly seen in women, particularly those who have been pregnant. In fact, research suggests that up to 60% of women who have given birth may experience some degree of abdominal separation. However, it's important to note that diastasis recti can also occur in men and in people who have never been pregnant.

There are several factors that can increase the risk of developing diastasis recti. Pregnancy is one of the most common risk factors, as the growing uterus can put pressure on the abdominal muscles and cause them to separate.

Other factors that may contribute to diastasis recti include:

- Obesity or carrying excess weight
- Multiple pregnancies or carrying a large baby
- Poor posture or improper lifting techniques
- Chronic coughing or straining

- Abdominal surgery or injury

It's worth noting that diastasis recti can also occur in people who are very physically fit and participate in activities such as weightlifting or certain yoga poses that put excessive strain on the abdominal muscles.

Diastasis recti and pregnancy

Diastasis recti is a common condition that occurs during pregnancy and can persist after childbirth. It is estimated that up to two-thirds of pregnant women develop some degree of diastasis recti. The growing uterus places pressure on the abdominal muscles, causing them to separate in the midline. This separation creates a gap between the left and right sides of the rectus abdominis muscle, which can lead to a bulging or protruding belly.

Diastasis recti during pregnancy can be caused by several factors, including hormonal changes, increased intra-abdominal pressure, and weakened abdominal muscles. As the uterus expands, it puts pressure on the abdominal wall and stretches the connective tissue that holds the rectus abdominis muscle together. Hormones such as relaxin, which is produced during pregnancy, can also contribute to the separation of the abdominal muscles by relaxing the connective tissue.

Other factors that can increase the risk of developing diastasis recti during pregnancy include carrying multiples, having a large baby, a previous pregnancy with diastasis recti, and a history of weak abdominal muscles. Additionally, women who are over the age of 35, have a high body mass index (BMI), or have excessive weight gain during pregnancy may also be at a higher risk.

It is important to note that while diastasis recti is common during pregnancy, it is not exclusive to pregnant women. Men, women who have never been pregnant, and even children can develop diastasis recti due to factors such as obesity, poor posture, or intense physical activity.

It is also important to understand that diastasis recti can affect women differently. Some women may not experience any symptoms, while others may have a noticeable bulge or protrusion in their abdomen. Additionally, some women may experience back pain or pelvic floor dysfunction, such as urinary incontinence, due to the weakened abdominal muscles.

Diastasis recti is typically diagnosed by a physical exam by a healthcare provider, who will check the separation of the abdominal muscles and the strength of the core muscles. Imaging tests, such as an ultrasound or MRI, may also be used to confirm the diagnosis or assess the severity of the condition.

While diastasis recti during pregnancy is common, there are steps that women can take to reduce their risk or prevent the condition from worsening. Engaging in regular exercise, such as prenatal yoga or pilates, can help strengthen the abdominal muscles and prevent further separation. It is also important to maintain good posture and avoid activities that place excess pressure on the abdomen, such as heavy lifting or crunches.

For women who do develop diastasis recti during pregnancy, postpartum exercises and physical therapy can help restore the strength and function of the abdominal muscles. In severe cases, surgery may be recommended to repair the separation of the abdominal muscles.

In summary, diastasis recti is a common condition that occurs when the abdominal muscles separate in the midline, often during pregnancy. While it can cause discomfort and other symptoms, there are steps that women can take to reduce their risk and prevent the condition from worsening.

With proper treatment and management, many women are able to recover from diastasis recti and restore the strength and function of their abdominal muscles.

Postpartum Diastasis Recti

Postpartum diastasis recti is a common condition that can occur in women during or after pregnancy. Diastasis recti is a separation of the rectus abdominis muscles, which run down the front of the abdomen and are often referred to as the "six-pack" muscles. This separation can cause a bulge or protrusion in the abdomen, and can be accompanied by other symptoms such as back pain, poor posture, and urinary incontinence.

During pregnancy, the uterus expands to accommodate the growing fetus, putting pressure on the abdominal muscles. This pressure can cause the rectus abdominis muscles to separate. In some cases, the separation may heal on its own after delivery, but in others, it may persist and require treatment.

It is estimated that up to 60% of women experience diastasis recti during pregnancy or postpartum. While it is more common in women who have had multiple pregnancies, it can occur in any woman.

The symptoms of postpartum diastasis recti can be distressing for new mothers, especially as they adjust to the physical changes that come with childbirth. Many women may feel self-conscious about the appearance of their abdomen, and may experience pain or discomfort when lifting or performing other physical activities.

Fortunately, there are non-surgical treatment options available for postpartum diastasis recti. These may include exercises and physical therapy to strengthen the abdominal muscles and improve posture. In some cases, a special support garment called an abdominal binder may be recommended to help support the abdominal muscles.

It is important to note that not all exercises are appropriate for women with postpartum diastasis recti, as certain movements may exacerbate the condition. A healthcare professional such as a physical therapist can work with the patient to develop a safe and effective exercise plan.

In some cases, surgical intervention may be necessary to correct postpartum diastasis recti. This may involve a procedure called a tummy tuck or abdominoplasty, which involves removing excess skin and tightening the abdominal muscles. However, surgery is typically only recommended in cases where non-surgical treatment options have been ineffective.

It is important for women to discuss any concerns about postpartum diastasis recti with their healthcare provider, as early intervention can lead to better outcomes. In addition to medical treatment, women can take steps to support their recovery, such as getting adequate rest, eating a healthy diet, and engaging in regular physical activity as recommended by their healthcare provider.

Obesity or carrying excess weight

Diastasis recti (DR) is a common condition that can affect both men and women, but it is more prevalent in women. Although pregnancy is a leading cause of DR, other factors can also lead to the condition, including obesity or carrying excess weight.

Obesity puts a significant amount of stress on the abdominal muscles, causing them to weaken and separate, leading to DR. The pressure of the excess weight can also cause a separation of the abdominal muscles, leading to a bulge in the midsection.

Carrying excess weight, even if not technically considered obese, can also increase the risk of DR. The excess weight places additional stress on the abdominal muscles, making them more susceptible to separating.

It's essential to note that DR can also occur in individuals who are of a healthy weight and have never been pregnant. In these cases, the condition is often the result of repetitive stress on the abdominal muscles, such as excessive heavy lifting or intense core exercises.

Regardless of the cause, DR can be a challenging condition to live with, as it can lead to discomfort and even pain in some cases. It can also cause a visible bulge in the midsection, which can lead to self-consciousness and body image concerns.

Fortunately, there are ways to prevent and treat DR, even for those who are obese or carrying excess weight. By making lifestyle changes, such as adopting a healthy diet and exercise routine, individuals can reduce their risk of DR and even improve their condition if they already have it.

Working with a physical therapist who specializes in DR can also be helpful. They can provide exercises and techniques that can help strengthen the abdominal muscles and close the separation. In some cases, surgery may be necessary to repair the separation fully, but this is typically only recommended in severe cases.

In conclusion, while obesity and carrying excess weight can increase the risk of developing diastasis recti, it's essential to note that anyone can develop the condition, regardless of their weight or pregnancy history. With proper prevention and treatment, individuals can live comfortably and confidently with diastasis recti.

Poor posture or improper lifting techniques

Diastasis recti, a condition that involves separation of the rectus abdominis muscles, can be caused by a variety of factors. One of the most common factors is poor posture, which can lead to muscle imbalances and weakness in the abdominal muscles. When the abdominal muscles are weakened, they may be more prone to separating during activities that place stress on the core, such as lifting heavy objects.

Improper lifting techniques can also contribute to the development of diastasis recti. When lifting heavy objects, it is important to engage the core muscles and lift with the legs, rather than using the back muscles to lift the object. Lifting with the back muscles can place excessive strain on the abdominal muscles, leading to separation.

Other factors that can increase the risk of developing diastasis recti include repetitive strain on the abdominal muscles, such as during certain exercises or activities, and hormonal changes, such as those that occur during pregnancy or menopause.

It is important to note that while poor posture and improper lifting techniques can contribute to the development of diastasis recti, they are not the only factors involved. It is also possible for diastasis recti to occur without any identifiable cause, especially in women who have had multiple pregnancies or who are carrying excess weight.

If you suspect that you may have diastasis recti, it is important to consult with a healthcare provider for an accurate diagnosis and appropriate treatment plan. Treatment may involve exercises to strengthen the abdominal muscles, as well as modifications to your daily activities to reduce strain on the core muscles. In some cases, surgery may be recommended to repair the separated muscles.

Chronic coughing or straining

Chronic coughing or straining can also contribute to the development of diastasis recti. People who have chronic coughing due to conditions such as asthma, bronchitis, or allergies may be at a higher risk for developing diastasis recti. Similarly, those who frequently strain during bowel movements due to constipation or other digestive issues may also be at a higher risk.

During coughing or straining, the increased pressure in the abdomen can cause the separation of the rectus abdominis muscles. This is because the muscles are not strong enough to withstand the pressure created by these actions. Over time, this can lead to the development of diastasis recti.

It is important to note that while chronic coughing or straining can contribute to the development of diastasis recti, they are not the sole cause. Other risk factors, such as pregnancy, obesity, and poor posture, can also play a role in the development of this condition. If you are experiencing symptoms of diastasis recti or are at risk for developing it, it is important to speak with a healthcare professional for evaluation and treatment.

Abdominal surgery or injury

Diastasis recti can also be caused by abdominal surgery or injury. In some cases, surgery or trauma can weaken the connective tissue of the abdominal muscles and cause them to separate. This can include surgeries such as c-sections or abdominal hernia repairs.

During a c-section, the abdominal muscles are cut through in order to access the uterus, and it can take several weeks or months for the muscles to fully heal and come back together. This healing process can be complicated if the muscles have already been weakened by pregnancy or other factors, potentially leading to diastasis recti.

Similarly, an abdominal hernia repair can weaken the abdominal muscles and potentially cause diastasis recti if the muscles are not properly repaired during surgery.

Trauma or injury to the abdominal area can also cause diastasis recti, particularly if it involves a significant impact to the area. In some cases, this can lead to a sudden separation of the abdominal muscles, but in others, it can cause a slow, gradual separation over time.

It's important to note that while abdominal surgery or injury can increase the risk of diastasis recti, not everyone who undergoes these experiences will develop the condition. Other factors, such as overall health and fitness levels, can also play a role in determining who is most at risk.

Chapter Five

Symptoms of Diastasis Recti

Diastasis recti is a condition in which the left and right sides of the rectus abdominis muscle – the "six-pack" muscle – separate along the linea alba, the connective tissue that runs down the center of the abdomen. This separation can cause a bulge in the midsection, sometimes described as a "pooch" or "mommy tummy."

In addition to the visible bulge, diastasis recti can cause a variety of symptoms, including:

1. Lower back pain: When the abdominal muscles are weakened and unable to provide adequate support for the spine, the lower back can become strained and painful.

2. Poor posture: A weakened core can cause a forward pelvic tilt and an increased curve in the lower back, leading to poor posture and potential pain and discomfort.

3. Digestive issues: Diastasis recti can impact the function of the abdominal muscles, which can affect digestion and bowel movements.

4. Weakness in the pelvic floor: The pelvic floor muscles work in conjunction with the abdominal muscles to support the core. When the abdominal muscles are weakened due to diastasis recti, it can also lead to weakness in the pelvic floor muscles.

5. Urinary incontinence: As a result of weakened pelvic floor muscles, urinary incontinence may occur.

6. Hernia: In severe cases, diastasis recti can lead to an abdominal hernia, which occurs when internal organs push through a weakened area of the abdominal wall.

It's important to note that not everyone with diastasis recti will experience symptoms, and some may have a mild case that doesn't require treatment. However, if you are experiencing any of these symptoms, it's important to speak with a healthcare provider to determine the best course of treatment.

Physical symptoms, including abdominal protrusion and back pain

Diastasis recti (DR) is a condition where the abdominal muscles separate due to a weakening of the connective tissue that holds them together. This separation can lead to a protruding belly, back pain, and other physical symptoms.

One of the most noticeable symptoms of DR is a bulging or protruding belly. This can occur even if the person is not pregnant or overweight. The bulge is caused by the separation of the rectus abdominis muscles, which are the muscles that run vertically down the middle of the abdomen. When these muscles separate, the connective tissue that holds them together (the linea alba) becomes stretched and weakened, allowing the abdominal contents to push forward.

In addition to a protruding belly, DR can also cause back pain. The weakened abdominal muscles are not able to provide as much support to the spine, which can lead to strain and discomfort. Other physical symptoms of DR may include constipation, bloating, and urinary incontinence.

It is important to note that not all people with DR will experience symptoms. In some cases, the separation of the abdominal muscles may be mild and not cause any noticeable physical changes or discomfort. However, even if there are no symptoms, it is still important to address DR to prevent it from getting worse over time.

If you suspect that you may have DR, it is important to see a healthcare provider for an evaluation. They can perform a physical exam to determine the severity of the condition and recommend appropriate treatment options.

Poor posture

Diastasis recti can cause poor posture due to the weakened abdominal muscles, which can result in a forward pelvic tilt and an increased curve in the lower back. This can lead to back pain and discomfort, as well as other related issues such as hip and knee pain, and difficulty with balance and stability.

In addition, poor posture can also lead to other health problems over time, including chronic headaches, neck pain, and shoulder pain. It can also affect breathing and digestion, as the weakened core muscles can impact the diaphragm and other internal organs.

It's important for individuals with diastasis recti to work with a healthcare professional or physical therapist to address any postural issues and develop an exercise program that will strengthen the core muscles and promote proper alignment. This may include exercises such as pelvic tilts, deep breathing techniques, and specific core strengthening exercises that target the transverse abdominis muscle.

Digestive issues

Diastasis recti can impact the function of the abdominal muscles, which can affect digestion and bowel movements. The separation of the rectus abdominis muscles can cause a loss of support for the internal organs, including the intestines. This can lead to problems with constipation, bloating, and other digestive issues. Additionally, the weakened abdominal muscles may not be able to properly contract and relax to facilitate bowel movements, leading to further complications. It is important to note that not all individuals with diastasis recti will experience digestive issues, but it is a potential symptom to be aware of.

Weakness in the pelvic floor:

Diastasis recti can weaken the pelvic floor muscles, which play a crucial role in supporting the bladder, uterus, and bowel. The pelvic floor muscles also aid in sexual function and help maintain continence.

When the abdominal muscles are weakened due to diastasis recti, it can cause the pelvic floor muscles to overcompensate, leading to an imbalance and potential dysfunction. This can result in symptoms such as urinary incontinence, pelvic pain, and painful intercourse. In some cases, a pelvic floor physical therapist may be able to help alleviate these symptoms by providing exercises to strengthen the pelvic floor muscles.

Urinary incontinence

Diastasis recti can also lead to urinary incontinence. This condition occurs when the pelvic floor muscles are unable to support the bladder and urethra, leading to the involuntary release of urine. This can happen during activities such as coughing, sneezing, laughing, or even exercising. In severe cases, it can occur during everyday activities such as standing up or walking. Urinary incontinence can significantly impact one's quality of life and lead to feelings of embarrassment or shame. It is important to seek medical attention if urinary incontinence is experienced.

Hernia

Diastasis recti can also lead to the development of a hernia. This occurs when the abdominal muscles are weakened to the point where internal organs, such as the intestines, can push through the weakened area of the abdominal wall. Hernias can be very painful and may require surgery to correct.

It's important to note that not all cases of diastasis recti will result in these symptoms, and the severity of the condition can vary from person to person. It's important to speak with a healthcare professional if you suspect you may have diastasis recti and are experiencing any of these symptoms.

Emotional symptoms, including body image issues and self-esteem

Diastasis recti can not only have physical symptoms, but can also have emotional symptoms as well. The physical changes in the body, such as a protruding abdomen and weakened core, can lead to body image issues and a decrease in self-esteem.

For many people, their self-image is closely tied to their physical appearance. When diastasis recti causes a protruding belly, it can be difficult for individuals to feel confident in their appearance. They may feel embarrassed or self-conscious about their body shape, and may avoid certain activities or clothing styles that draw attention to their midsection.

In addition to body image issues, diastasis recti can also cause feelings of frustration or helplessness. Individuals may feel frustrated that they cannot perform certain exercises or movements that they once could, and may feel helpless in trying to improve their condition.

These emotional symptoms can have a significant impact on overall well-being and quality of life. It is important for individuals with diastasis recti to address not only the physical symptoms, but also the emotional ones. Seeking support from loved ones, speaking with a therapist, or joining a support group can all be helpful in managing these emotional symptoms.

It is also important to remember that diastasis recti is a common condition, and does not define a person's worth or value. By focusing on self-care and seeking support, individuals with diastasis recti can improve their physical and emotional well-being and regain their confidence and self-esteem.

The Do's and Don'ts of Diastasis Recti

Diastasis recti is a condition that can be treated with various methods, including physical therapy and exercise. However, it's important to know what activities to avoid to prevent worsening the condition. Here are some do's and don'ts of diastasis recti:

Do's:

1. Consult with a healthcare professional: The first step in treating diastasis recti is to speak with a healthcare professional. They can recommend appropriate treatment options and advise you on the do's and don'ts of managing the condition.

2. Perform appropriate exercises: Certain exercises can help strengthen the core muscles and improve diastasis recti. These exercises include pelvic tilts, gentle crunches, and modified planks.

3. Use proper posture: Maintaining good posture throughout the day can help improve diastasis recti. Stand up straight, and avoid slouching or leaning forward.

4. Use proper lifting techniques: When lifting heavy objects, bend at the knees and keep your core engaged. Avoid lifting objects that are too heavy for you.

5. Wear supportive clothing: Wearing compression garments or a supportive belt can help improve diastasis recti and prevent worsening of the condition.

Don'ts:

1. Avoid crunches and sit-ups: These exercises can strain the abdominal muscles and worsen diastasis recti. Instead, focus on exercises that strengthen the core muscles without putting undue stress on them.

2. Avoid heavy lifting: Heavy lifting can put additional strain on the weakened abdominal muscles, making diastasis recti worse. If you must lift something heavy, engage your core and use proper lifting techniques.

3. Don't engage in high-impact exercises: Activities such as running or jumping can put too much stress on the abdominal muscles and worsen diastasis recti. Instead, try low-impact exercises like walking, swimming, or yoga.

4. Avoid twisting movements: Twisting motions can put additional strain on the weakened abdominal muscles and worsen diastasis recti. Instead, try exercises that focus on stabilization and strengthening.

5. Don't ignore symptoms: If you experience symptoms such as abdominal pain or back pain, don't ignore them. Consult with a healthcare professional to determine the best course of treatment.

In conclusion, diastasis recti can be treated with various non-surgical methods, including exercise and physical therapy. However, it's important to know what activities to avoid to prevent worsening the condition. By following the do's and don'ts of diastasis recti, you can manage the condition and improve your quality of life.

Chapter Six

Diagnosis of Diastasis Recti

Diastasis recti can be diagnosed through a physical examination by a healthcare provider or a fitness professional trained in identifying the condition. During the examination, the provider will have the individual lie down on their back with their knees bent and feet on the floor. They will then place their fingers along the midline of the abdomen and ask the individual to perform a small crunch or raise their head and shoulders slightly off the ground. This allows the provider to feel for any separation of the abdominal muscles and determine the severity of the condition.

In some cases, imaging studies such as ultrasound or magnetic resonance imaging (MRI) may be used to confirm the diagnosis and assess the extent of the separation. However, these imaging studies are not typically necessary unless there is a concern for a more severe underlying condition, such as a hernia.

It is important for individuals to seek medical evaluation if they suspect they may have diastasis recti, as other conditions such as hernias may have similar symptoms and require different treatment. A healthcare provider can provide a proper diagnosis and develop an appropriate treatment plan.

How diastasis recti

is

diagnosed

Diastasis recti can often be diagnosed through a physical exam by a healthcare provider. During the exam, the healthcare provider will ask the patient to lie on their back with their knees bent and their feet flat on the floor. The provider will then place their fingers at the center of the patient's abdomen, just above the belly button, and ask the patient to raise their head and shoulders off the ground.

If the abdominal muscles have separated, the healthcare provider will be able to feel a gap between the muscles, and may be able to determine the width and depth of the separation. The healthcare provider may also use a measuring tape to measure the distance between the abdominal muscles.

In some cases, imaging tests such as an ultrasound or MRI may be used to confirm the diagnosis and assess the severity of the separation. These tests can provide a more detailed view of the abdominal muscles and the degree of separation.

It is important for individuals who suspect they may have diastasis recti to seek evaluation and diagnosis from a healthcare provider. Proper diagnosis can help ensure appropriate treatment and management of the condition.

The role of healthcare professionals

Diastasis recti is a condition that can significantly impact the quality of life of those affected by it. Seeking professional medical advice is often necessary to properly diagnose and treat the condition.

A primary care physician or OB-GYN can typically diagnose diastasis recti during a physical exam. The healthcare professional will ask the patient to lie on their back with their knees bent and feet flat on the floor. The examiner will then place their fingers just above the belly button and ask the patient to perform a crunch-like movement. If the examiner feels a gap between the two sides of the rectus abdominis muscle, diastasis recti may be diagnosed.

In some cases, imaging tests such as ultrasound or MRI may be used to confirm the diagnosis and assess the severity of the condition.

If the healthcare professional suspects that another underlying condition is contributing to the diastasis recti, further testing or referral to a specialist may be necessary. For example, if a hernia is suspected, a surgical consult may be needed.

It is important for healthcare professionals to be knowledgeable about diastasis recti and its potential impact on patients' health and well-being. They can provide education and support to help patients manage the condition, and can refer them to physical therapists or other specialists for treatment as needed.

Tests and assessments used to diagnose the condition

There are several tests and assessments that healthcare professionals may use to diagnose diastasis recti. These include:

1. Physical examination: The healthcare professional will feel the abdominal muscles and check for the separation between the muscles. They may ask the patient to perform exercises to assess muscle strength.

2. Ultrasound: An ultrasound can be used to confirm the separation between the abdominal muscles and assess the extent of the separation.

3. CT scan or MRI: These imaging tests can provide more detailed information about the separation between the abdominal muscles and help identify any other underlying conditions.

4. Electromyography (EMG): This test measures the electrical activity in the muscles and can help assess muscle function.

5. Pelvic floor assessment: If the patient is experiencing pelvic floor dysfunction, a pelvic floor assessment may be conducted to evaluate muscle strength and function.

It's important to note that not all cases of diastasis recti require medical intervention. In some cases, physical therapy exercises and lifestyle modifications may be sufficient to address the condition. However, if the separation is severe, surgery may be required to repair the abdominal muscles.

Chapter Seven

Treatment Options for Diastasis Recti

Diastasis recti is a condition that causes a separation of the rectus abdominis muscles, which run down the front of the abdomen. While it is a common condition, affecting up to 60% of women postpartum, it can also occur in men and non-pregnant women. The good news is that diastasis recti can often be treated through a combination of exercises, lifestyle modifications, and in some cases, surgery.

Here are some of the most common treatment options for diastasis recti:

1. Physical therapy: A physical therapist can create a customized exercise program to strengthen the muscles of the abdomen, back, and pelvic floor. This may include exercises such as kegels, pelvic tilts, and bridges.

2. Core strengthening exercises: Specific exercises can help to strengthen the abdominal muscles and reduce the separation between them. These exercises may include crunches, planks, and bird dogs.

3. Weight management: Carrying excess weight can put extra strain on the abdominal muscles and exacerbate diastasis recti. Maintaining a healthy weight through diet and exercise can help to alleviate symptoms.

4. Good posture: Poor posture can increase the strain on the abdom-

inal muscles, exacerbating diastasis recti. Proper posture, including sitting up straight and engaging the core muscles, can help to alleviate symptoms.

5. Supportive garments: Some women find relief by wearing a supportive garment such as a postpartum belly band or compression shorts.

6. Surgery: In severe cases, surgery may be necessary to repair the separation between the abdominal muscles. This is typically a last resort and is only considered when other treatment options have been exhausted.

It is important to note that not all cases of diastasis recti require treatment, and for some individuals, the separation between the abdominal muscles may improve on its own over time. However, for those experiencing pain, discomfort, or other symptoms, seeking medical attention is recommended.

In addition to the above treatment options, there are some exercises and movements to avoid with diastasis recti. These include traditional sit-ups, crunches, and planks, which can put too much strain on the weakened abdominal muscles. Instead, modified versions of these exercises or alternative exercises that don't put as much pressure on the abdomen may be recommended.

Overall, the treatment of diastasis recti is highly individualized, and the best course of action will depend on the severity of the condition, the underlying cause, and the patient's individual needs and goals. Consulting with a healthcare professional, such as a physical therapist or physician, is recommended to develop a treatment plan that is safe and effective.

Non-surgical treatment options, including exercises and physical therapy

Diastasis recti, a condition characterized by the separation of the rectus abdominis muscles, can be treated non-surgically through exercises and physical therapy. These options are aimed at strengthening the core muscles and closing the gap between the separated muscles. Here are some non-surgical treatment options for diastasis recti:

1. Core-strengthening exercises: Exercises that target the core muscles, including the transverse abdominis, pelvic floor, and obliques, can help improve the strength and stability of the abdominal muscles. These exercises include planks, squats, lunges, bridges, and pelvic tilts.

2. Physical therapy: Physical therapy can help to improve posture, alignment, and muscle strength. Physical therapists can work with patients to develop a personalized exercise program that targets their specific needs and goals. They may also use modalities such as ultrasound or electrical stimulation to assist in muscle re-education and contraction.

3. Belly binding: Wearing a belly binder or compression garment can help to support the abdominal muscles and reduce the gap between the separated muscles. This can provide additional support during exercise or activities that require core engagement.

4. Postural adjustments: Making adjustments to posture and body mechanics can help to prevent further separation of the abdominal muscles. Practicing good posture and avoiding activities that require heavy lifting or straining can help to prevent the condition from worsening.

5. Breathing techniques: Proper breathing techniques can help to engage the deep core muscles, including the transverse abdominis and pelvic floor. These muscles play a key role in stabilizing the spine and supporting the abdominal muscles.

It is important to note that while these non-surgical options can be effective for some patients, they may not be appropriate for everyone. In some cases, surgery may be necessary to repair the separation of the abdominal muscles. It is important to consult with a healthcare professional to determine the best course of treatment for your specific needs and goals.

Surgical treatment options

Diastasis recti, a condition where the abdominal muscles separate and cause a protruding belly, can sometimes require surgical intervention if non-surgical options are not effective. Surgical treatment options for diastasis recti include abdominoplasty, also known as a tummy tuck, and hernia repair.

Abdominoplasty involves removing excess skin and fat from the abdomen and tightening the abdominal muscles to restore a more toned appearance. During the procedure, the surgeon makes an incision across the lower abdomen, lifts the skin and fat, and tightens the muscles with sutures. The excess skin and fat are then removed, and the incision is closed with sutures or surgical tape.

Hernia repair is another surgical option for diastasis recti. In severe cases, the separation of the abdominal muscles can lead to an abdominal hernia, which occurs when internal organs push through a weakened area of the abdominal wall. Hernia repair surgery involves closing the opening in the abdominal wall and strengthening the weakened area with mesh.

While surgery can be effective in treating diastasis recti, it is important to note that it is a major procedure and should be carefully considered. It also carries the risks of any surgical procedure, including bleeding, infection, and adverse reactions to anesthesia.

Surgical treatment options for diastasis recti are typically reserved for cases where non-surgical options, such as physical therapy and exercise, have been unsuccessful in improving symptoms. It is important to consult with a qualified healthcare professional to determine the best course of treatment for individual cases of diastasis recti.

A

bdominoplasty

Surgical treatment options for diastasis recti include abdominoplasty, also known as a tummy tuck. Abdominoplasty is a major surgical procedure that involves removing excess skin and fat from the abdomen and tightening the muscles in the abdominal wall.

During an abdominoplasty procedure, the surgeon makes an incision across the lower abdomen, just above the pubic area. The skin and fat are lifted away from the abdominal muscles, and the muscles are pulled together and stitched in place, effectively narrowing the gap caused by diastasis recti.

Excess skin and fat are then removed, and the remaining skin is stretched downward to create a smoother, tighter appearance. The incision is then closed with stitches or surgical tape.

Abdominoplasty is a highly invasive procedure and requires a longer recovery time than non-surgical treatments. Patients may need to take several weeks off work and avoid strenuous activity during the recovery period.

While abdominoplasty can effectively treat diastasis recti and provide a more toned appearance, it is important to note that it is a major surgical procedure and carries the same risks and potential complications as any other surgery. These can include infection, bleeding, blood clots, and poor wound healing.

It is also important to note that abdominoplasty is not recommended for everyone. Candidates should be in good overall health, have realistic expectations for the outcome of the surgery, and be committed to maintaining a healthy lifestyle after the procedure. Patients who smoke or have underlying health conditions that could increase the risk of complications may not be good candidates for the surgery.

Overall, while surgical options like abdominoplasty can be effective for treating diastasis recti, they should be carefully considered and discussed with a qualified healthcare professional. Non-surgical treatment options, including exercises and physical therapy, are often recommended as a first-line approach and can be effective for many patients.

H

ernia repair.

Hernia repair is a surgical procedure that involves the repair of a hernia, which is a condition where an organ or tissue bulges through a weak spot in the surrounding muscle or connective tissue. Hernias can occur in various parts of the body, but the most common areas are the abdominal wall, groin, and diaphragm.

There are two main types of hernias: inguinal hernias, which occur in the groin area, and ventral hernias, which occur in the abdominal wall. Both types of hernias can be repaired using surgical techniques.

The surgical treatment of hernias typically involves repairing the weakened area of the muscle or connective tissue, either by sewing it together or by using a mesh patch to reinforce the area. The surgical approach may be open or minimally invasive, depending on the type and size of the hernia.

Open hernia repair involves making an incision in the area of the hernia, and then repairing the weakened area of the muscle or connective tissue. This approach may be used for larger hernias or for hernias that have recurred after a previous repair. In some cases, a laparoscopic or robotic-assisted approach may be used, which involves making several small incisions and using a tiny camera and special instruments to repair the hernia.

The use of a mesh patch is common in hernia repair, as it helps to reinforce the weakened area and prevent a recurrence of the hernia. The mesh patch can be made of various materials, including synthetic materials or animal tissue.

Recovery from hernia repair surgery typically involves a period of rest and limited physical activity, followed by a gradual return to normal activities over several weeks. Pain medication and other supportive measures may be prescribed to manage pain and discomfort during the recovery period.

Complications of hernia repair surgery are rare but can include infection, bleeding, and damage to surrounding tissues or organs. In some cases, a recurrence of the hernia may occur despite the surgical repair.

Overall, hernia repair surgery is a safe and effective treatment option for those with hernias, and can provide relief from symptoms and prevent complications associated with this condition.

The role of nutrition and lifestyle changes in treatment

Diastasis recti, a condition where the abdominal muscles separate, can be treated through various non-surgical methods such as physical therapy and exercise. However, nutrition and lifestyle changes can also play a significant role in the treatment of diastasis recti. Making small changes in your lifestyle and diet can help support the healing process and reduce the risk of worsening the condition.

One important aspect of nutrition when dealing with diastasis recti is ensuring that you are consuming enough protein. Protein is necessary for the growth and repair of muscles, and adequate intake can help support the healing process. Some excellent sources of protein include lean meats, fish, eggs, and legumes.

Another important aspect of nutrition is hydration. Proper hydration is necessary for the body to function properly and can also help support the healing process. Drinking adequate amounts of water and avoiding sugary drinks can be helpful in this regard.

In addition to nutrition, making lifestyle changes can also be beneficial in the treatment of diastasis recti. One of the most important changes you can make is to avoid activities that may exacerbate the condition, such as heavy lifting, repetitive twisting, and sit-ups. Instead, focus on low-impact exercises that engage the core muscles without putting undue stress on them, such as yoga, Pilates, or swimming.

Improving your posture can also be helpful in the treatment of diastasis recti. Slouching or leaning forward can put pressure on the abdominal muscles and exacerbate the condition. Instead, focus on sitting or standing up straight, with your shoulders back and your pelvis slightly tilted forward.

Stress management techniques can also be helpful in the treatment of diastasis recti. Stress can cause tension in the body, which can lead to muscle tension and strain. Practicing relaxation techniques such as deep breathing, meditation, or yoga can help alleviate tension and support the healing process.

In summary, while non-surgical methods such as exercise and physical therapy are the mainstays of diastasis recti treatment, nutrition and lifestyle changes can also play a significant role. By consuming adequate amounts of protein and staying hydrated, avoiding activities that may exacerbate the condition, improving your posture, and managing stress, you can support the healing process and reduce the risk of worsening the condition.

Chapter Eight

Exercises for Healing Diastasis Recti

Hip Bridge Lifts

Hip bridge lifts, also known as glute bridges, are a popular exercise used to strengthen the muscles in the glutes, hamstrings, and lower back. They can also be helpful for individuals with diastasis recti, as they engage the core muscles without putting too much pressure on the abdominal wall.

To perform a hip bridge lift, follow these steps:

1. Lie on your back with your knees bent and feet flat on the ground, hip-width apart.
2. Place your arms by your sides with your palms facing down.
3. Engage your core muscles by drawing your navel in towards your spine.
4. Squeeze your glutes and lift your hips off the ground until your body forms a straight line from your shoulders to your knees.
5. Hold for a few seconds, then slowly lower your hips back down to the ground.
6. Repeat for 10-15 reps.

When performing hip bridge lifts, it's important to focus on using your glutes to lift your hips, rather than relying on your lower back muscles. You should also avoid arching your back or tilting your pelvis too much, as this can put extra pressure on the abdominal wall.

It's also possible to modify hip bridge lifts to make them more challenging or to target different muscle groups. For example, you can try single-leg hip bridges to increase the intensity, or you can place a resistance band around your thighs to engage your outer hip muscles.

Overall, hip bridge lifts can be a great exercise for individuals with diastasis recti, as they can help strengthen the core and lower body without aggravating the condition. As always, it's important to consult with a healthcare professional before starting any new exercise program, especially if you have a pre-existing condition like diastasis recti.

Candle Exhales

Candle exhales, also known as diaphragmatic breathing or belly breathing, is a deep breathing technique that can help improve lung capacity and reduce stress and anxiety. The technique is called "candle exhales" because the exhale is performed as if blowing out a candle.

To perform the candle exhale technique:

1. Sit or lie down comfortably in a quiet place.
2. Place one hand on your chest and the other hand on your belly.
3. Take a slow, deep breath in through your nose, focusing on filling your belly with air rather than your chest.
4. Hold the breath for a few seconds.

5. Exhale slowly through your mouth, as if blowing out a candle, feeling your belly deflate.

6. Repeat for several breaths, focusing on the sensation of your hands rising and falling with your breaths.

By focusing on breathing into your belly, you engage the diaphragm muscle, which helps to expand the lungs and promote relaxation. Candle exhales can also be used as a relaxation technique during times of stress or anxiety. With regular practice, this technique can help to reduce tension and promote a sense of calm.

It's important to note that while candle exhales can be helpful, they should not be used as a replacement for medical treatment for respiratory or mental health conditions. If you experience any persistent symptoms or difficulty breathing, it's important to consult with your healthcare provider.

Heel Slides

Heel slides are a simple yet effective exercise for strengthening the abdominal muscles and helping to close the separation of the rectus abdominis that can occur with diastasis recti.

To perform heel slides, follow these steps:

1. Lie on your back with your knees bent and feet flat on the ground.

2. Place your hands on your abdomen, just above your belly button.

3. Inhale deeply, and as you exhale, engage your abdominal muscles by drawing your belly button toward your spine. This is also known as activating your core.

4. Slowly slide one foot away from your body while keeping your

knee bent, while at the same time sliding your opposite hand up your thigh.

5. Return your leg and hand back to their starting position and repeat on the other side.

6. Repeat for several repetitions on each side, aiming for 10-15 repetitions per side.

Remember to keep your core engaged throughout the exercise and move slowly and deliberately, avoiding any jerky or sudden movements. This exercise can be modified as needed to accommodate your fitness level and any physical limitations you may have. It is important to consult with a healthcare professional before beginning any exercise program, especially if you have diastasis recti or other medical conditions.

Single Leg Extensions

Single leg extensions are an exercise that can help strengthen the core muscles and alleviate the symptoms of diastasis recti. This exercise targets the lower abdominal muscles, which are often weakened in people with diastasis recti.

To perform single leg extensions:

1. Lie flat on your back with your knees bent and feet flat on the ground.

2. Tighten your abdominal muscles and press your lower back into the floor.

3. Slowly lift one leg off the ground, keeping your knee bent.

4. Straighten the lifted leg and hold it in the air for a few seconds.

5. Slowly lower the leg back to the starting position.
6. Repeat with the other leg.
7. Aim to complete 10-15 repetitions on each leg.

It's important to keep your core muscles engaged throughout the exercise and avoid any movements that cause your abdominal muscles to bulge outwards. If you experience any pain or discomfort while performing single leg extensions, stop the exercise and consult with your healthcare provider.

Single Leg Lifts

Single leg lifts are an exercise that can help strengthen the abdominal muscles and reduce the appearance of diastasis recti. This exercise targets the lower abdominal muscles, which are often weakened in people with diastasis recti.

To perform single leg lifts, follow these steps:

1. Lie on your back with your knees bent and your feet flat on the floor.
2. Tighten your abdominal muscles by pulling your belly button towards your spine.
3. Lift one leg off the ground, keeping the knee bent and the foot flat.
4. Hold for a few seconds, then lower the leg back down.
5. Repeat with the other leg.

Make sure to keep your back flat on the ground and avoid arching it during the exercise. If you feel any discomfort or pain, stop the exercise immediately and consult with a healthcare professional.

To make the exercise more challenging, you can try straightening your leg as you lift it off the ground, or adding ankle weights. It's important to start with a few repetitions and gradually increase the number as you build strength. Aim to do 10-15 repetitions on each leg.

Remember that single leg lifts are just one exercise that can help with diastasis recti. It's important to also incorporate other exercises and treatments, such as pelvic tilts, kegels, and physical therapy, as recommended by a healthcare professional.

Single Leg Marches

Single Leg Marches is a beneficial exercise for people with diastasis recti. It strengthens the transverse abdominis, which is essential for healing diastasis recti. The transverse abdominis is a deep muscle in the abdomen that acts as a corset, supporting the abdominal wall and helping to stabilize the spine. Strengthening this muscle can help reduce the gap in the abdominal muscles, which is a key factor in diastasis recti.

To perform the Single Leg Marches exercise:

1. Lie on your back with your knees bent and feet flat on the ground.
2. Place your hands on your belly, just above your belly button.
3. Take a deep breath in and exhale slowly, engaging your deep abdominal muscles by pulling your belly button towards your spine.
4. Lift one foot off the ground, straightening the leg, while main-

taining engagement in your deep abdominal muscles.

5. Hold the leg up for a few seconds, then slowly lower it back down to the ground.

6. Repeat with the other leg.

7. Continue alternating legs, aiming for 10-12 repetitions on each side.

It is important to maintain proper form and alignment during this exercise. Be sure to keep your spine in a neutral position, avoid arching your back, and keep your core muscles engaged throughout the movement. If you experience any pain or discomfort, stop the exercise and consult with a healthcare professional before continuing.

Alternating Heel Taps

Alternating heel taps is an exercise commonly recommended to address diastasis recti, a separation of the rectus abdominis muscles. This exercise can be done in a variety of positions, including lying on the back, seated, or standing.

To perform alternating heel taps while lying on the back, follow these steps:

1. Lie on your back with your knees bent and your feet flat on the ground.

2. Place your hands on your stomach, just above your belly button.

3. Take a deep breath in, and as you exhale, gently engage your abdominal muscles by pulling your belly button in towards your spine.

4. While keeping your abdominal muscles engaged, lift one foot off the ground and tap your heel on the floor.

5. Lower your foot back to the ground, and repeat on the other side.

6. Continue to alternate tapping your heels for 10-15 repetitions on each side.

It's important to avoid straining or bulging the abdominal muscles during this exercise, as this can make diastasis recti worse. Keep your movements slow and controlled, and focus on using your deep core muscles to stabilize your spine.

Alternating heel taps can help to improve core strength and stability, which can in turn help to reduce the symptoms of diastasis recti. It's important to work with a qualified healthcare professional to develop a personalized exercise program that addresses your specific needs and goals.

Reverse Crunches

Reverse crunches are an exercise that targets the lower abdominals, or rectus abdominis, and can be effective in improving core strength and stability.

Here's how to perform reverse crunches:

1. Lie flat on your back with your legs bent and your feet flat on the ground.

2. Place your hands behind your head or to the sides of your body.

3. Lift your legs off the ground, bending your knees so that they form a 90-degree angle.

4. Slowly lift your hips off the ground, bringing your knees towards your chest.

5. Pause at the top of the movement, squeezing your abs.

6. Slowly lower your hips and legs back down to the starting position.

It's important to maintain proper form while performing reverse crunches. Avoid jerking or swinging your legs, as this can put unnecessary strain on your lower back. Instead, focus on using your abdominal muscles to lift your hips off the ground. Start with a few reps and gradually increase as your core strength improves.

Reverse crunches can be a great addition to your workout routine, especially if you're looking to strengthen your core and improve overall stability. Remember to always listen to your body and consult with a healthcare professional before beginning any new exercise program.

Straight Leg Reverse Crunches

Straight Leg Reverse Crunches are an excellent exercise for strengthening the lower abdominal muscles, which can help improve diastasis recti. This exercise targets the rectus abdominis, which is the muscle that runs vertically down the front of the abdomen and is often weakened with diastasis recti.

To perform straight leg reverse crunches:

1. Lie on your back with your legs straight up in the air, perpendicular to the ground. Place your hands on the floor next to your hips.

2. Keeping your legs straight, lift your hips off the floor and towards

your chest. Use your lower abdominal muscles to lift your hips, rather than using momentum.

3. Lower your hips back down to the starting position, hovering just above the ground.

4. Repeat for 10-15 repetitions.

To increase the challenge of this exercise, you can add ankle weights or hold a light dumbbell between your feet. Be sure to engage your lower abdominal muscles throughout the exercise and avoid using momentum to lift your hips.

Modified Knee Drops

Modified Knee Drops is an exercise that can help strengthen the transverse abdominis muscles, which can help in the recovery of diastasis recti. It is a gentle exercise that can be done by anyone, regardless of fitness level or experience.

To perform Modified Knee Drops, follow these steps:

1. Lie on your back with your knees bent and feet flat on the ground.

2. Place a small ball or rolled-up towel between your knees.

3. Slowly lower both knees to one side, keeping your shoulders on the ground.

4. Hold for a few seconds and then return to the starting position.

5. Repeat on the other side.

It is important to keep your core engaged throughout the exercise and avoid using momentum to move your legs. You should also avoid lowering your legs too far if it causes discomfort or pain.

This exercise can be done daily as part of a larger exercise routine or as a standalone exercise. As with any exercise program, it is important to consult with a healthcare professional before starting, especially if you have any pre-existing conditions or injuries.

Knee Drops

Knee drops are a common exercise used to target the abdominal muscles, particularly the transverse abdominis muscle, which can help to improve diastasis recti. This exercise is relatively simple and can be done by anyone, regardless of their fitness level or experience.

To perform knee drops, follow these steps:

1. Lie flat on your back with your knees bent and your feet flat on the floor.

2. Place your arms out to the sides with your palms facing down.

3. Slowly lower both knees to one side, keeping your feet in contact with the ground. Only lower your knees as far as you can while maintaining contact between your feet and the ground.

4. Hold the stretch for a few seconds, then slowly raise your knees back up to the starting position.

5. Repeat the exercise on the other side, lowering your knees to the opposite side.

6. Continue to alternate sides, performing 10-12 repetitions on each

side.

It's important to keep your movements slow and controlled throughout the exercise. Focus on engaging your core muscles, particularly your transverse abdominis, as you lower and raise your legs.

If you experience any discomfort or pain during the exercise, stop immediately and consult with a healthcare professional.

Forearm Plank Hip Dips

Forearm plank hip dips are a challenging exercise that targets the core, specifically the obliques. This exercise involves getting into a forearm plank position and then slowly dipping your hips to one side, engaging your oblique muscles, before bringing them back up to center and repeating on the other side.

Here's how to perform forearm plank hip dips:

1. Begin by getting into a forearm plank position, with your elbows directly under your shoulders and your forearms on the ground.
2. Engage your core and keep your spine straight.
3. Slowly dip your hips to the right, keeping your core engaged and your back straight. Lower your hips as far as you can without touching the ground.
4. Hold for a few seconds before raising your hips back up to center.
5. Repeat on the left side, dipping your hips to the left and then raising them back up to center.
6. Continue alternating sides for 10-12 repetitions.

Forearm plank hip dips can be modified by dropping to your knees instead of staying on your toes, and by lowering your hips for a smaller range of motion. As you progress, you can increase the range of motion by dipping your hips lower to the ground.

It's important to remember to engage your core throughout the entire exercise and to keep your movements slow and controlled to prevent any strain on your lower back. If you experience any pain or discomfort, stop the exercise and consult with a medical professional.

Incorporating forearm plank hip dips into your regular exercise routine can help to strengthen your core, improve your posture, and increase overall stability and balance.

Side Plank Hold

The side plank hold is a core-strengthening exercise that targets the obliques, which are muscles on the sides of the abdomen. It also works the glutes, shoulders, and back muscles.

To perform a side plank hold:

1. Start by lying on your side with your legs straight and feet stacked on top of each other.

2. Prop yourself up on your elbow and forearm, with your elbow directly below your shoulder.

3. Lift your hips off the ground, forming a straight line from your head to your feet.

4. Engage your core muscles and hold the position for 30 seconds to 1 minute.

5. Lower your hips back down to the ground and switch to the other side.

6. Repeat for 2-3 sets on each side.

It's important to maintain proper form during the side plank hold. Keep your body in a straight line, avoiding sagging or bending at the waist. Keep your shoulders relaxed and your neck in a neutral position. If you experience any pain or discomfort, stop the exercise and consult with a healthcare professional.

Incorporating side plank holds into your fitness routine can help improve core stability, balance, and posture. It's a versatile exercise that can be modified to suit different fitness levels, such as by holding the plank from the knees rather than the feet.

Pelvic Brace

Pelvic brace is a type of exercise that can help individuals with diastasis recti to strengthen their core muscles and reduce the severity of the condition. It is also known as "belly breathing" or "transverse abdominal bracing".

The exercise involves contracting the transverse abdominal muscles, which are located deep in the abdomen, below the rectus abdominis muscles. These muscles act like a corset around the waist, supporting the internal organs and providing stability to the spine.

To perform the pelvic brace exercise:

1. Lie on your back with your knees bent and feet flat on the floor.

2. Place your hands on your lower abdomen, just below your belly button.

3. Take a deep breath in through your nose, filling your lungs with air.

4. As you exhale through your mouth, gently draw your belly button towards your spine, tightening the muscles in your lower abdomen.

5. Hold the contraction for a few seconds, then release and inhale.

6. Repeat for several repetitions, aiming for 10 to 15 repetitions per set.

It is important to perform the pelvic brace exercise correctly to ensure that the transverse abdominal muscles are being targeted. Avoid holding your breath or tensing other muscles, such as the glutes or thigh muscles, as this can reduce the effectiveness of the exercise.

The pelvic brace exercise can be performed as a standalone exercise or as part of a wider exercise program designed to address diastasis recti. It is important to consult with a healthcare professional or a qualified fitness instructor before starting any exercise program, especially if you have diastasis recti or other underlying health conditions. They can provide guidance on how to perform exercises correctly and safely, as well as recommend modifications or alternative exercises if needed.

Toe Dips

Toe dips are an exercise that targets the core muscles, specifically the transverse abdominis, which can help alleviate symptoms of diastasis recti. This exercise is simple, low-impact, and can be done at home without any equipment.

To perform toe dips, follow these steps:

1. Lie on your back with your knees bent and your feet flat on the floor.

2. Tighten your abdominal muscles and press your lower back into the floor.

3. Slowly lower one foot toward the floor, keeping your knee bent.

4. As you lower your foot, exhale and draw your belly button toward your spine, engaging your transverse abdominis.

5. Hold the position for a few seconds, then return to the starting position.

6. Repeat the movement with your other foot.

Start with 5-10 repetitions on each side, gradually increasing the number of reps as you feel stronger. As you progress, you can also try extending one leg while lowering the other, or lifting your head and shoulders off the floor for an added challenge.

Toe dips are a great exercise for anyone looking to strengthen their core and alleviate symptoms of diastasis recti. However, it's important to remember that this exercise alone may not be enough to fully heal diastasis recti. It's important to work with a healthcare professional, such as a physical therapist, to develop a comprehensive treatment plan that addresses all aspects of the condition.

Transverse Abdominis Engagement

The transverse abdominis is a deep muscle in the abdomen that plays a key role in stabilizing the core and supporting the spine. When this muscle is weak, it can contribute to conditions such as low back pain and diastasis recti.

To engage the transverse abdominis, try the following exercise:

1. Lie on your back with your knees bent and feet flat on the floor.
2. Place your hands on your lower abdomen, just above your pelvic bone.
3. Take a deep breath in and let your belly expand.
4. As you exhale, gently draw your navel in towards your spine, as if you are trying to zip up a tight pair of pants.
5. Hold this contraction for a few seconds, then release and repeat.
6. Be sure to keep breathing normally throughout the exercise.

It may take some practice to fully engage the transverse abdominis, as it is a deep muscle that is often underused. As you get more comfortable with this exercise, try incorporating it into your daily routine, such as during periods of sitting or when lifting heavy objects. Over time, this can help to improve your core stability and reduce your risk of injury.

Building a Diastasis Recti Workout Circuit

If you have been diagnosed with diastasis recti, it is important to work on healing and strengthening your core muscles. A diastasis recti workout circuit can be a great way to target those muscles and improve your overall fitness.

Here are some exercises you can incorporate into your workout circuit:

1. Toe taps: Lie on your back with your knees bent and feet on the floor. Lift one foot off the ground and tap your toe on the floor. Alternate legs for 30 seconds.

2. Plank: Start in a push-up position with your arms straight and hands shoulder-width apart. Lower your forearms to the ground and hold your body in a straight line from head to toe for 30 seconds.

3. Hip bridge: Lie on your back with your knees bent and feet on the ground. Lift your hips off the ground, squeezing your glutes and engaging your core muscles. Hold for 30 seconds.

4. Modified knee drops: Lie on your back with your knees bent and feet on the floor. Drop your knees to one side, keeping your shoulders on the ground. Bring your knees back to center and repeat on the other side for 30 seconds.

5. Forearm plank hip dips: Start in a forearm plank position with your elbows on the ground and your body in a straight line from head to toe. Dip your hips to one side and then the other, making sure to keep your core engaged. Repeat for 30 seconds.

6. Single leg lifts: Lie on your back with your knees bent and feet on the ground. Lift one foot off the ground and straighten your leg. Lower your leg back down and repeat on the other side for 30 seconds.

7. Side plank hold: Lie on your side with your elbow on the ground and your body in a straight line from head to toe. Hold for 30 seconds and then switch sides.

8. Transverse abdominis engagement: Stand with your feet shoul-

der-width apart and engage your transverse abdominis muscle by drawing your belly button in towards your spine. Hold for 30 seconds.

9. Alternating heel taps: Lie on your back with your knees bent and feet on the floor. Lift one foot off the ground and tap your heel on the floor. Alternate legs for 30 seconds.

10. Knee drops: Lie on your back with your knees bent and feet on the floor. Drop both knees to one side, keeping your shoulders on the ground. Bring your knees back to center and repeat on the other side for 30 seconds.

Remember to listen to your body and start slowly. Aim to complete 2-3 rounds of the circuit, resting for 30-60 seconds between each exercise. As your strength and endurance improve, you can increase the number of rounds or the length of each exercise.

Chapter Nine

Living with Diastasis Recti

Living with diastasis recti can be challenging, but with proper treatment and self-care, it is possible to manage the condition and live a fulfilling life.

Here are some tips for living with diastasis recti:

1. Follow a healthy diet: Eating a healthy diet can help manage diastasis recti symptoms by promoting healing and reducing inflammation. Focus on nutrient-dense foods, such as fruits, vegetables, lean proteins, and whole grains.

2. Maintain good posture: Poor posture can worsen diastasis recti symptoms, so be sure to practice good posture by sitting and standing up straight, keeping your shoulders relaxed, and engaging your core muscles.

3. Avoid heavy lifting: Heavy lifting can strain the abdominal muscles and exacerbate diastasis recti symptoms. If you need to lift something heavy, be sure to use proper lifting techniques and engage your core muscles.

4. Stay active: Exercise can be beneficial for managing diastasis recti symptoms, but be sure to choose exercises that are safe for your condition. Consult with a physical therapist or personal trainer who is knowledgeable about diastasis recti to create a safe and

effective exercise plan.

5. Wear supportive clothing: Wearing supportive clothing, such as a maternity support belt, can help support the abdominal muscles and alleviate symptoms.

6. Seek support: Living with diastasis recti can be challenging, both physically and emotionally. Don't be afraid to seek support from friends, family, or a support group. You can also consult with a mental health professional to address any emotional challenges you may be experiencing.

7. Consider surgery: In some cases, surgery may be necessary to repair diastasis recti. If you are considering surgery, be sure to consult with a qualified surgeon and thoroughly research the procedure and recovery process.

Living with diastasis recti requires patience, persistence, and a willingness to make lifestyle changes. With the right care and support, it is possible to manage the condition and live a healthy, fulfilling life.

Coping with the physical and emotional impact of the condition

Diastasis recti can have a significant impact on both physical and emotional well-being. Coping with the condition requires a multi-faceted approach that includes physical therapy, lifestyle modifications, and emotional support.

One of the most important aspects of coping with diastasis recti is learning to manage physical symptoms. Physical therapy can be an effective way to strengthen the core muscles and reduce the severity of symptoms. Physical therapists can teach patients how to perform exercises that are safe and effective for their specific condition.

It is also important to make lifestyle changes that can reduce the severity of symptoms. Maintaining a healthy weight, avoiding heavy lifting, and practicing good posture can all help reduce the strain on the abdominal muscles.

In addition to physical symptoms, diastasis recti can also have an emotional impact. Many people with the condition experience body image issues and low self-esteem. It can be helpful to talk to a therapist or support group to work through these feelings and develop coping strategies.

Finally, it is important to have a strong support system when coping with diastasis recti. This may include family members, friends, or a support group. It can also be helpful to work with a healthcare provider who is knowledgeable about the condition and can provide guidance and support.

While living with diastasis recti can be challenging, there are many effective ways to manage the condition and improve overall well-being. By working with healthcare providers, making lifestyle changes, and seeking emotional support, individuals with diastasis recti can reduce symptoms and improve their quality of life.

Tips for managing symptoms and improving quality of life

Diastasis recti can have a significant impact on quality of life, both physically and emotionally. However, there are several ways to manage the symptoms and improve overall well-being.

1. Exercise and physical therapy: As discussed earlier, exercises and

physical therapy can help improve the strength and tone of the abdominal muscles, which can alleviate many of the physical symptoms of diastasis recti.

2. Mind-body techniques: Mind-body techniques such as yoga, meditation, and deep breathing can help manage stress and improve overall well-being. These techniques can also help improve posture and alignment, which can alleviate physical symptoms.

3. Nutrition: Eating a healthy, balanced diet can help promote overall health and well-being. This can also help manage weight, which can reduce strain on the abdominal muscles.

4. Supportive garments: Supportive garments such as abdominal binders or compression garments can help support the abdominal muscles and alleviate physical symptoms.

5. Emotional support: Dealing with the emotional impact of diastasis recti can be challenging. Seeking support from friends, family, or a mental health professional can be helpful in managing the emotional impact of the condition.

6. Avoiding certain activities: Certain activities, such as heavy lifting or high-impact exercise, can exacerbate the symptoms of diastasis recti. Avoiding these activities or modifying them to reduce strain on the abdominal muscles can be helpful.

7. Seeking medical treatment: In some cases, surgical treatment may be necessary to repair diastasis recti. Consulting with a medical professional can help determine the best course of treatment.

Managing the symptoms of diastasis recti may require a combination of approaches. However, with the right tools and support, it is possible to manage the physical and emotional impact of the condition and improve overall quality of life.

Chapter Ten

Personal stories from individuals living with diastasis recti

Tracy

's Story

I'm feeling frustrated and overwhelmed lately, and it's all because of this condition called diastasis recti. I never even heard of it until my doctor diagnosed me with it after my third pregnancy. Apparently, it's common for women who have had multiple pregnancies, and it means that my abdominal muscles have separated, causing my belly to bulge out and creating all sorts of problems.

It's been a few months since my diagnosis, and I've been trying everything to fix it. I've been doing these exercises that my doctor recommended, like pelvic tilts and heel slides, but it doesn't seem to be helping much. I still have this bulge, and I feel so self-conscious about it.

What's worse is that I'm experiencing back pain and poor posture, which I never had before. I feel like my body is failing me, and it's affecting my confidence and self-esteem. My husband tells me that I look beautiful no matter what, but it's hard to believe him when I don't even feel comfortable in my own skin.

I'm trying to stay positive and focus on the things that I can control. I've been trying to eat healthier and exercise regularly, and I'm doing my best to take care of myself. But some days, it feels like it's all for nothing.

I know that there are worse things in life, but it's hard not to feel defeated by this condition. I'm grateful for the support of my husband and family, but I wish that more people understood what I'm going through.

Anyway, I'll keep pushing through and trying to stay positive. Hopefully, things will start to improve soon.

Natasha's Story

It's been a few months since I gave birth to my baby girl, and I've been experiencing some unusual symptoms that I can't ignore anymore. I've been noticing a separation between my abdominal muscles, which has made it difficult to engage my core during workouts. I did some research, and it seems like I have a condition called diastasis recti.

I didn't even know what diastasis recti was until now. Apparently, it's a common condition that can happen during pregnancy, especially if you carry your baby low like I did. The pressure from the baby can cause the muscles to separate, leaving a gap between them. It's also more common if you've had multiple pregnancies or if you're over the age of 35, which I am.

I remember during my last trimester, my belly was so huge that I could barely move around. The pressure was intense, and I would often feel out of breath or like I couldn't get comfortable no matter how I positioned myself. I didn't think much of it at the time, but now I'm wondering if that's when the separation began.

I've been doing some exercises to try to close the gap between my abdominal muscles, but it's been slow progress. I know it takes time, but it's frustrating to feel like I'm not making much of a difference. Plus, it's hard to find the time to work out with a newborn baby to take care of.

I'm also dealing with some postpartum depression, which is making it harder to stay motivated and keep a positive attitude. I've been feeling self-conscious about my body and struggling with my self-esteem. It's hard to see all these new moms on social media bouncing back to their pre-pregnancy bodies when I feel like I'm stuck in this awkward in-between phase.

I know I need to be patient with myself and focus on healing both physically and mentally. I'm trying to eat a balanced diet and get as much rest as I can, but it's not easy. I'm grateful to have a supportive partner in my husband, who has been helping me take care of the baby and encouraging me to take time for myself.

I'm hoping that with time, I'll start to see some improvements in my body and in my mood. It's hard to remember that these things take time and that there's no one "right" way to recover from pregnancy and childbirth. I just have to keep reminding myself that I'm doing the best I can and that I'm not alone in this.

Steph's Story

Today was my six-week postpartum check-up, and my doctor told me I have diastasis recti. I had never heard of this condition before, and I was immediately filled with worry and anxiety.

My pregnancy and delivery were both difficult, and now it seems that I have this additional issue to deal with. My doctor explained that diastasis recti is a separation of the abdominal muscles that can occur during pregnancy due to the pressure put on the abdominal wall. This can cause a protruding belly and other unpleasant symptoms.

Thinking back on my delivery, I remember the intense pressure and strain that I felt in my abdomen. I had to push for hours, and it felt like my body was being torn apart. Now, I realize that this pressure likely contributed to my diastasis recti.

My doctor gave me some exercises to do to help heal my abdominal muscles, but I know it will be a long road. It's frustrating because I want to get back to my pre-pregnancy body, but I know that I need to be patient and take things slow.

It's also difficult because I have a newborn to take care of, and it can be challenging to find time to fit in the exercises and self-care that I need. But I know that I need to prioritize my health so that I can be the best mother possible for my baby.

I'm feeling overwhelmed and scared, but I know that I'm not alone. I've heard of other women who have had diastasis recti and have been able to overcome it with time and patience. I'm hopeful that I can do the same.

Nicole's Story

I never thought I'd be the one to have a horrendous childbirth experience, but that's exactly what happened. My labor went on for what felt like an eternity - 36 hours to be exact. It was excruciating and I felt like giving up multiple times.

After all that pain and struggle, I was overjoyed to finally hold my baby girl in my arms. But as the days went on, I started to feel like something was wrong. My abdomen felt weak and my back was constantly sore. I chalked it up to the physical toll of childbirth and assumed it would get better with time.

But as time went on, my symptoms didn't improve. I started to notice a bulge in my abdomen that wouldn't go away, no matter how much I exercised or watched my diet. It wasn't until I saw a specialist that I learned I had diastasis recti, a condition where the abdominal muscles separate during pregnancy or childbirth.

I was devastated to learn that my body had gone through so much trauma during childbirth that it left me with a lasting condition. It was tough to come to terms with, but I knew I had to take action to manage my symptoms.

My doctor recommended physical therapy and specific exercises to help strengthen my core muscles and improve my posture. It was a long road, but with consistent effort and the support of my loved ones, I slowly started to see progress.

Even though it's been a difficult journey, I'm grateful for the lessons I've learned along the way. I've come to appreciate the strength and resilience of my body, even in the face of immense physical and emotional stress. And I'm reminded every day of the incredible blessing that is my daughter, who made it all worth it.

Anna's Story

I never imagined my childbirth experience would be so intense. I was well overdue, and my baby weighed a whopping 12.3 pounds! The delivery was a long and grueling process, and I thought it would never end.

After the delivery, I was in shock and completely exhausted. I barely had the energy to hold my newborn baby, let alone take care of myself. Over the next few weeks, I started experiencing some strange symptoms, like a bulging belly and back pain.

I went to my doctor, who diagnosed me with diastasis recti. I had never heard of this condition before, but I learned that it was caused by the separation of the abdominal muscles during pregnancy and childbirth. The size of my baby likely contributed to the severity of my case.

I was devastated. As a new mother, I already felt overwhelmed and now I had to deal with this as well. My doctor suggested some exercises and physical therapy to help strengthen my core and alleviate some of the symptoms.

It was a long road to recovery, but I eventually started to see some improvement. I had to make some lifestyle changes and take things slow, but I was determined to get better.

I realized that I wasn't alone in my struggle with diastasis recti. Many women experience this condition, and it can be a challenging journey. But with the right support and resources, it is possible to manage the symptoms and improve quality of life.

So if you're going through something similar, don't give up hope. There are options available to you and a community of people who understand what you're going through.

Jane's Story

I cannot believe how exhausted I am. I just gave birth to my beautiful baby boy, but it was one of the most difficult experiences of my life. He was 10 days overdue and weighed a not funny 11 pounds! The labor was long, and the delivery was traumatic.

After the delivery, I noticed that my stomach had a bulge that didn't seem to go away. I was also experiencing lower back pain and had difficulty sitting up straight. My doctor diagnosed me with diastasis recti, which meant that my abdominal muscles had separated during pregnancy and childbirth.

I was devastated to learn about this condition, as I had never heard of it before. I felt like my body had failed me, and I was worried that I would never fully recover. However, my doctor reassured me that with proper treatment and exercise, I could heal and regain my strength.

I started attending physical therapy sessions to help me retrain my muscles and close the separation. My therapist showed me exercises that focused on engaging my core muscles and slowly building up my strength. I also started wearing an abdominal binder to support my muscles and help them heal.

It has been a challenging journey, but I am starting to see progress. My stomach bulge has reduced, and my back pain has decreased. I am also feeling more confident in my ability to recover and regain my strength.

Despite the difficulties, I am grateful for my beautiful baby boy and for the support of my loved ones. I know that I still have a long road ahead of me, but I am determined to heal and become stronger than ever.

Chapter Eleven

Preventing Diastasis Recti

Diastasis recti is a condition that can occur for a variety of reasons, including pregnancy, obesity, and abdominal surgery. While it may not be entirely preventable in all cases, there are steps that can be taken to reduce the risk of developing diastasis recti.

Here are some tips for preventing diastasis recti:

1. Maintain a healthy weight: Obesity and carrying excess weight are risk factors for diastasis recti. Maintaining a healthy weight through a balanced diet and regular exercise can help reduce the risk of developing this condition.

2. Practice good posture: Poor posture can contribute to diastasis recti by putting extra pressure on the abdominal muscles. Be mindful of your posture throughout the day and try to sit and stand with your shoulders back and your spine aligned.

3. Use proper lifting techniques: Lifting heavy objects improperly can strain the abdominal muscles and contribute to diastasis recti. When lifting heavy objects, be sure to use your legs and not your back, and engage your core muscles to help support your spine.

4. Avoid activities that strain the abdominal muscles: Chronic coughing or straining, such as during bowel movements, can weaken the abdominal muscles and increase the risk of diastasis

recti. If you are prone to these activities, talk to your healthcare provider about ways to manage them.

5. Exercise regularly: Regular exercise can help strengthen the abdominal muscles and reduce the risk of diastasis recti. However, it's important to avoid exercises that may make the condition worse, such as traditional sit-ups or crunches. Instead, focus on exercises that engage the transverse abdominal muscles, such as pelvic tilts and planks.

6. Seek treatment for existing conditions: If you have a pre-existing condition, such as a hernia or chronic cough, that puts extra strain on your abdominal muscles, seek treatment for that condition to reduce the risk of developing diastasis recti.

7. Consult with a healthcare provider: If you are pregnant or have recently given birth, consult with your healthcare provider about ways to reduce your risk of developing diastasis recti. They may be able to recommend exercises or other preventative measures to help keep your abdominal muscles strong.

Overall, taking care of your body through healthy habits and regular exercise can help reduce the risk of developing diastasis recti. If you are concerned about your risk for this condition, talk to your healthcare provider about ways to prevent it or manage any existing symptoms.

How to prevent diastasis recti during pregnancy and childbirth

Diastasis recti is a common condition that occurs when the rectus abdominis muscles separate during pregnancy or childbirth. While it is not always possible to prevent diastasis recti, there are steps that women can take to reduce their risk of developing the condition.

Here are some tips for preventing diastasis recti during pregnancy and childbirth:

1. Exercise regularly: Regular exercise can help keep the abdominal muscles strong and improve core strength, which can reduce the risk of diastasis recti. It is important to choose exercises that are safe for pregnancy and to consult with a healthcare provider before starting any new exercise program.

2. Maintain good posture: Good posture can help support the abdominal muscles and reduce the risk of diastasis recti. Women should try to sit and stand up straight, avoid slouching, and use proper lifting techniques.

3. Avoid excessive weight gain: Excessive weight gain during pregnancy can put extra strain on the abdominal muscles and increase the risk of diastasis recti. Women should aim to gain a healthy amount of weight during pregnancy, as recommended by their healthcare provider.

4. Practice safe childbirth techniques: During childbirth, women can reduce the risk of diastasis recti by practicing safe pushing techniques. This can include using breathing techniques and avoiding holding their breath while pushing.

5. Wear supportive clothing: Wearing supportive clothing, such as a maternity support belt, can help support the abdominal muscles during pregnancy and reduce the risk of diastasis recti.

6. Manage constipation: Chronic constipation can put extra strain

on the abdominal muscles and increase the risk of diastasis recti. Women should aim to maintain regular bowel movements by staying hydrated, eating a fiber-rich diet, and exercising regularly.

7. Consult with a healthcare provider: Women should consult with their healthcare provider about their risk of diastasis recti and any steps they can take to reduce their risk. Women with a history of diastasis recti or other abdominal issues may be at higher risk and may need additional support and guidance.

By following these tips, women can reduce their risk of developing diastasis recti and promote a healthy pregnancy and childbirth.

Exercises and lifestyle changes to help prevent the condition

Diastasis recti is a condition that occurs when the two halves of the rectus abdominis muscle separate, leading to a visible bulge in the midline of the abdomen. While this condition is more commonly seen in women during and after pregnancy, it can also affect men and women who engage in certain activities that place excessive strain on the abdominal muscles.

Fortunately, there are several exercises and lifestyle changes that can help prevent diastasis recti.

Here are a few examples:

1. Pelvic tilts: Pelvic tilts can help strengthen the abdominal muscles and prevent them from separating. To perform a pelvic tilt, lie on your back with your knees bent and feet flat on the floor. Tighten your abdominal muscles and press your lower back into the floor, holding for a few seconds before releasing.

2. Kegels: Kegel exercises can help strengthen the pelvic floor muscles, which play a key role in supporting the abdominal muscles. To perform Kegels, contract your pelvic floor muscles as if you were trying to stop the flow of urine. Hold the contraction for a few seconds before releasing.

3. Planks: Planks are an effective exercise for strengthening the core muscles, including the rectus abdominis. To perform a plank, get into a push-up position with your forearms on the ground and your body in a straight line. Hold the position for as long as you can, focusing on keeping your core engaged.

4. Squats: Squats are another effective exercise for strengthening the core muscles and preventing diastasis recti. To perform a squat, stand with your feet hip-width apart and your toes pointing forward. Bend your knees and lower your body, keeping your back straight and your core engaged.

In addition to exercise, there are also some lifestyle changes that can help prevent diastasis recti. For example, maintaining good posture can help prevent excessive strain on the abdominal muscles. It is also important to avoid activities that place excessive strain on the abdominal muscles, such as heavy lifting or straining during bowel movements.

In conclusion, diastasis recti is a condition that can be prevented with the right exercise and lifestyle habits. By incorporating exercises that strengthen the abdominal muscles and adopting healthy lifestyle habits, you can reduce your risk of developing this condition and improve your overall quality of life. As always, it is important to consult with your healthcare provider before starting any new exercise program.

The importance of seeking medical advice and support

Diastasis recti is a common condition that can affect both men and women, and it is important to seek medical advice and support if you suspect you may be experiencing symptoms. While there are many non-surgical treatment options available, it is important to have a healthcare professional evaluate your condition to determine the best course of action.

If you are experiencing symptoms of diastasis recti, such as abdominal protrusion or back pain, it is important to seek medical attention. Your healthcare provider may recommend non-surgical treatment options, such as exercises or physical therapy, to help strengthen your abdominal muscles and alleviate symptoms.

It is also important to maintain a healthy lifestyle, including a balanced diet and regular exercise, to help prevent the development of diastasis recti. During pregnancy, practicing good posture and avoiding heavy lifting can also help reduce your risk of developing the condition.

In addition to seeking medical advice and making lifestyle changes, it can also be helpful to connect with others who have experienced diastasis recti. Support groups and online forums can provide a space to share experiences, ask questions, and receive emotional support.

Remember, it is important to prioritize your health and seek the support you need to manage and overcome diastasis recti. With the right treatment and support, it is possible to improve symptoms and maintain a high quality of life.

Chapter Twelve

Supporting Loved Ones with Diastasis Recti

Diastasis recti is a common condition that affects many people, but often women who have recently given birth. Although it is not a life-threatening condition, it can cause discomfort, pain, and a host of other symptoms. If you have a loved one who is dealing with diastasis recti, there are several things you can do to support them and help them manage their symptoms.

1. Listen and be empathetic: Diastasis recti can be a challenging and isolating experience. It's essential to listen to your loved one and offer empathy and support. Acknowledge their feelings and frustrations and offer words of encouragement. Let them know that you are there for them and that you understand how difficult this can be.

2. Help with daily tasks: If your loved one is experiencing pain or discomfort, they may have trouble completing everyday tasks. Offer to help with childcare, housework, or other responsibilities to give them time to rest and recover.

3. Encourage exercise: Although strenuous exercise is not recommended for those with diastasis recti, gentle exercise can help strengthen the core muscles and alleviate symptoms. Encourage your loved one to talk to their healthcare provider about safe exercise options.

4. Help them find resources: There are many resources available for those with diastasis recti, including physical therapists, online support groups, and educational materials. Help your loved one find the resources they need to manage their symptoms effectively.

5. Be patient: Diastasis recti can take time to heal, and the process can be frustrating for your loved one. Be patient and understanding and offer your support throughout their recovery journey.

6. Encourage healthy habits: Eating a healthy diet and getting enough sleep are essential for overall health and can also help manage diastasis recti symptoms. Encourage your loved one to make healthy choices and offer to join them in these habits.

In summary, supporting a loved one with diastasis recti involves being empathetic, helping with daily tasks, encouraging safe exercise, finding resources, being patient, and encouraging healthy habits. By offering your support, you can help your loved one manage their symptoms and feel more confident and comfortable in their recovery journey.

How to support a partner, family member, or friend with the condition

Diastasis recti can be a difficult condition to live with, and those affected by it may benefit greatly from the support of their loved ones. If someone you know is struggling with diastasis recti, there are several ways you can support them and help improve their quality of life. Here are some tips:

1. Listen: First and foremost, it's important to be a good listener. Encourage your loved one to talk about their experiences, their feelings, and any challenges they are facing. Be empathetic and non-judgmental, and offer your support in whatever way you can.

2. Help with daily tasks: Diastasis recti can make it difficult for individuals to perform certain activities, such as lifting heavy objects or carrying groceries. Offer to help with these tasks when you can, or assist with other daily activities that may be challenging.

3. Encourage exercise: Exercise can be an effective way to strengthen the core muscles and reduce the symptoms of diastasis recti. Encourage your loved one to talk to their healthcare provider about safe and effective exercises they can do, and offer to exercise with them for motivation and support.

4. Offer healthy food choices: Eating a healthy diet can also be beneficial for those with diastasis recti. Offer to prepare healthy meals together or provide healthy food options to support your loved one's nutrition goals.

5. Be patient and understanding: Living with diastasis recti can be frustrating and challenging, and progress may not always be immediate. Be patient with your loved one and offer your understanding and support throughout their journey.

6. Educate yourself: Educating yourself about diastasis recti and the challenges it presents can also be beneficial in supporting your loved one. Read up on the condition and be prepared to offer information and resources to help them in their journey.

7. Seek professional support: Encourage your loved one to seek the support of a healthcare provider or specialist who can offer additional guidance and treatment options. Offer to accompany them to appointments and help with any necessary arrangements.

In conclusion, supporting a loved one with diastasis recti can be challenging, but it is also a meaningful way to show your care and compassion. With patience, empathy, and support, you can help your loved one manage their symptoms and improve their quality of life.

Tips for providing emotional support and practical assistance

Diastasis recti, a condition characterized by a separation of the rectus abdominis muscles, can have a significant impact on an individual's physical and emotional wellbeing. If someone you know is living with diastasis recti, providing them with emotional support and practical assistance can make a big difference in their quality of life.

Here are some tips for supporting loved ones with diastasis recti:

1. Be a good listener: People living with diastasis recti may experience frustration, anxiety, and even depression due to the physical and emotional impact of the condition. Be there to listen and provide a safe space for your loved one to express their feelings.

2. Offer practical assistance: Individuals with diastasis recti may struggle with activities of daily living, such as carrying heavy objects, lifting children, or bending over. Offer to help with these tasks or find ways to make them easier, such as using a stroller or carrying groceries in a backpack.

3. Provide emotional support: Living with diastasis recti can be isolating and may lead to feelings of low self-esteem and body image issues. Encourage your loved one to seek professional help if necessary and offer words of encouragement and validation.

4. Educate yourself: Learn more about diastasis recti, including the causes, symptoms, and treatment options. This can help you bet-

ter understand what your loved one is going through and provide more effective support.

5. Be patient: Recovery from diastasis recti can take time, and progress may be slow. Be patient with your loved one and avoid pressuring them to "bounce back" too quickly.

6. Help them find resources: Connect your loved one with health-care professionals, such as physical therapists and personal trainers who specialize in diastasis recti. You can also provide them with information about support groups, online forums, and other resources that may be helpful.

7. Celebrate progress: Celebrate your loved one's successes, no matter how small they may seem. Whether it's successfully completing a physical therapy session or feeling more confident in their body, acknowledge and celebrate progress along the way.

By providing emotional support and practical assistance, you can help your loved one with diastasis recti cope with the challenges of the condition and improve their quality of life.

The importance of education and understanding

Diastasis recti can be a challenging condition to understand and live with, not just for the person affected, but also for their loved ones. If you have a partner, family member, or friend who is living with diastasis recti, it's important to educate yourself on the condition and provide support and understanding.

One of the most important things you can do to support someone with diastasis recti is to listen to their concerns and validate their experiences.

Diastasis recti can be a source of physical and emotional discomfort, and it can be helpful for the person to have someone to talk to about their experiences.

You can also provide practical assistance to help them manage the condition. This might include helping them with household chores, childcare, or running errands, especially during times when they are experiencing more severe symptoms.

Encouraging healthy habits can also be beneficial for someone with diastasis recti. This might include helping them with meal planning and preparation, encouraging them to engage in regular exercise (with the guidance of a medical professional), and helping them to prioritize sleep and stress management.

It's important to remember that diastasis recti is a physical condition that can have emotional and psychological effects. Supporting your loved one emotionally and providing a safe space for them to talk about their experiences can be incredibly helpful.

Finally, it's important to understand that there is no one-size-fits-all approach to managing diastasis recti. Each person's experience with the condition is unique, and it's important to respect their choices and decisions regarding their own care. Encouraging them to seek medical advice and supporting them in their treatment decisions can help them to manage the condition more effectively.

Chapter Thirteen

Looking Forward with Diastasis Recti

Diastasis recti can be a frustrating and challenging condition to live with, but there are many ways to manage the symptoms and improve quality of life. It's important to remember that while the condition can be difficult to deal with, it is not life-threatening and there are treatment options available.

If you are living with diastasis recti, here are some tips to help you look forward and take control of your condition:

1. Stay active: Regular exercise and physical activity can help to strengthen the abdominal muscles and improve core stability. However, it's important to avoid exercises that may exacerbate the condition or cause further damage. Consult with a physical therapist or fitness professional who is knowledgeable about diastasis recti to create a safe and effective exercise routine.

2. Seek support: Living with diastasis recti can be emotionally and mentally challenging. Seek out support from family, friends, or a support group to help you cope with the condition. A mental health professional may also be able to provide additional support and coping strategies.

3. Make lifestyle changes: Certain lifestyle factors, such as poor posture, improper lifting techniques, and obesity, can contribute to the development of diastasis recti. Making changes to these factors

can help to prevent further damage and improve symptoms.

4. Consider treatment options: Depending on the severity of the condition, surgery may be necessary to repair the abdominal muscles. However, non-surgical options such as physical therapy and exercise can also be effective in managing symptoms and improving core strength.

5. Practice self-care: It's important to take care of yourself and prioritize self-care when living with diastasis recti. This can include getting enough sleep, eating a balanced and nutritious diet, and engaging in stress-reducing activities such as yoga or meditation.

In conclusion, living with diastasis recti can be challenging, but with the right support and management strategies, it is possible to improve symptoms and regain control. It's important to work with healthcare professionals and loved ones to develop a personalized treatment plan and prioritize self-care in order to look forward and live a healthy and fulfilling life.

Current research and advancements in treatment options

Diastasis recti is a common condition that affects many individuals, particularly women during pregnancy and postpartum. While non-surgical treatment options such as exercises and physical therapy are often effective, some individuals may require surgical intervention, such as a hernia repair or abdominoplasty, to achieve the desired outcome.

Recent advancements in surgical techniques have led to improved outcomes and reduced risks for individuals with diastasis recti. For example, endoscopic surgery, which involves small incisions and the use of a camera to guide the surgical instruments, can lead to faster recovery times and reduced scarring compared to traditional open surgery.

In addition to surgical advancements, research is also being conducted on the effectiveness of new non-surgical treatment options. One such option is the use of a specialized abdominal brace that applies pressure to the abdominal muscles, encouraging them to come back together. Another option is the use of neuromuscular electrical stimulation, which involves the use of small electrical currents to stimulate the abdominal muscles and promote healing.

It is important to note that more research is needed in these areas to fully understand their effectiveness and potential risks.

In terms of prevention, research is also being conducted on the role of lifestyle factors such as diet and exercise in reducing the risk of developing diastasis recti. For example, maintaining a healthy weight and engaging in regular physical activity can help support the abdominal muscles and reduce the risk of injury.

Overall, while diastasis recti can have a significant impact on an individual's quality of life, there is hope for those living with the condition. Advances in both surgical and non-surgical treatment options, as well as continued research on prevention and management, are providing new avenues for improved outcomes and increased well-being.

The role of advocacy and awareness in improving outcomes for individuals with diastasis recti

Diastasis recti (DR) is a common condition that affects many individuals, particularly women who have been pregnant. While there are non-surgical and surgical treatment options available for DR, many individuals still struggle to receive proper diagnosis and treatment due to lack of awareness and advocacy.

Advocacy efforts for diastasis recti have been ongoing for several years, with many organizations and individuals working to raise awareness about the condition and improve outcomes for those affected. One such organization is the Diastasis Recti Association (DRA), a non-profit organization that seeks to provide support and education to individuals with DR, as well as to healthcare professionals who may encounter the condition in their practice.

The DRA provides a range of resources for individuals with DR, including information on exercise and physical therapy, nutrition and lifestyle changes, and surgical options. They also offer a directory of healthcare professionals who are knowledgeable about DR and its treatment, making it easier for individuals to find the support they need.

In addition to organizations like the DRA, there are also many individuals who are speaking out about their experiences with DR and advocating for better care and treatment options. Social media has been a particularly powerful tool for these individuals, allowing them to connect with others who are going through similar experiences and share their stories with a wider audience.

One such advocate is Leah Keller, creator of the online program The Dia Method, which provides a series of exercises and techniques to help heal DR. Keller has been a vocal advocate for DR awareness and education, and has worked to empower individuals with the tools and knowledge they need to manage their condition.

Another advocate is Jenna Dalton, founder of the blog and social media account Ab and Core Rehab, which provides information and resources on DR, as well as exercises and techniques to help manage the condition.

Dalton has also shared her own personal experience with DR, and has worked to break down stigma and shame surrounding the condition.

Advocacy and awareness efforts have also led to increased research and advancements in treatment options for DR. In recent years, there has been a growing body of research on the effectiveness of exercise and physical therapy for DR, as well as on the potential benefits of surgical options like abdominoplasty.

One promising area of research is the use of ultrasound imaging to better diagnose and monitor DR. While ultrasound has traditionally been used for imaging during pregnancy, it is now being used to visualize the abdominal muscles and measure the degree of separation in cases of DR. This technology has the potential to provide more accurate and precise diagnosis and treatment options for individuals with the condition.

In conclusion, advocacy and awareness are essential for improving outcomes for individuals with diastasis recti. By raising awareness about the condition, providing education and resources for both individuals and healthcare professionals, and promoting research and advancements in treatment options, we can improve the lives of those affected by this common and often misunderstood condition.

Chapter Fourteen

Living with Diastasis Recti

Diastasis recti is a condition in which the abdominal muscles separate, causing a protrusion of the belly. This separation can occur as a result of pregnancy, weight gain, or abdominal surgery. Living with diastasis recti can be challenging, as the condition can cause physical discomfort and emotional distress. However, with the right support and management strategies, individuals with diastasis recti can improve their quality of life.

One of the most important things for individuals with diastasis recti is to seek medical advice and support. A healthcare professional can provide an accurate diagnosis, as well as recommend appropriate treatment options. This may include physical therapy, specialized exercises, or even surgery, depending on the severity of the condition.

In addition to seeking medical advice, there are a number of lifestyle changes that can help manage the symptoms of diastasis recti. One of the most effective strategies is to engage in regular exercise, particularly exercises that focus on strengthening the core muscles. Physical therapists can provide personalized exercise plans that target the specific needs of individuals with diastasis recti.

It is also important for individuals with diastasis recti to maintain good posture and avoid activities that put strain on the abdominal muscles, such as heavy lifting or certain types of exercise. Wearing supportive garments, such as abdominal binders or compression garments, can also help manage symptoms and provide additional support.

Emotional support is also crucial for individuals with diastasis recti. The condition can cause body image issues and self-esteem problems, particularly in women who have experienced the condition as a result of pregnancy. Seeking out support from friends, family, or a therapist can be helpful in managing these emotional challenges.

Finally, advocacy and awareness can play an important role in improving outcomes for individuals with diastasis recti. By educating others about the condition and advocating for better treatment options, individuals with diastasis recti can help reduce the stigma and improve access to care for those living with the condition.

In conclusion, living with diastasis recti can be challenging, but with the right support and management strategies, individuals with the condition can improve their quality of life. Seeking medical advice, engaging in regular exercise, maintaining good posture, seeking emotional support, and advocating for better treatment options are all important steps in managing the symptoms of diastasis recti and improving outcomes for those living with the condition.

Chapter Fifteen

Frequently Asked Questions.

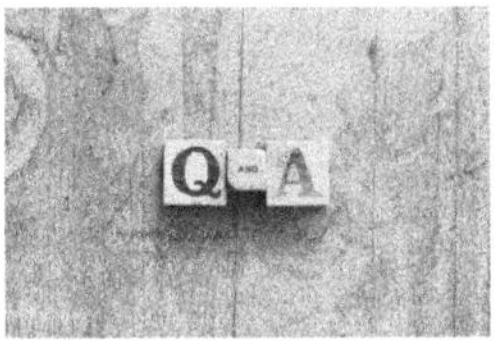

How do I know if I have diastasis recti?

There are a few things to look for that may indicate you have diastasis recti. First, you can try the Diagnostic Test for Diastasis Recti from Tupler Technique. Second, are you able to place more than two fingers inside your abdominal muscles at the midline? Third, does your abdomen protrude when you cough or sneeze? Fourth, can you only feel your abdominal muscles contracting when you place your hand on the outside of your abdomen? Lastly, when you lie down and press on your stomach, does your upper stomach bulge out away from your fingers? If you answered yes to any of these, you may have diastasis recti. It's also important to know that diastasis recti isn't just a "pregnancy thing." Men, women, and children of all ages and sizes can have diastasis recti. The condition is also relatively common in post-partum women and in obese individuals.

What happens if diastasis recti goes untreated?

If diastasis recti—the separation of the abdominal muscles—goes untreated, a number of things may happen. For one, because the abdominal muscles are not working as they should, it can lead to back pain. In addition, untreated diastasis recti may cause urination issues, as well as constipation. Additionally, hernias may develop, and women may experience pelvic floor prolapse. All of these issues can be extremely uncomfortable and may negatively impact quality of life. If you think you may have diastasis recti, be sure to see a doctor so that you can get the treatment you need.

Does diastasis recti go away?

Diastasis recti is a separation of the abdominal muscles that can occur during pregnancy. The abdominal muscles expand during pregnancy to accommodate the growing fetus, and the connective tissue between the muscles stretches. This can cause the muscles to separate, and diastasis recti can occur. After the baby is born, the abdominal muscles will contract and the connective tissue will start to heal. The separation of the muscles will start to improve, but it may take several months for the muscles to fully heal. For some women, the separation may not heal completely and may require further treatment. Most women will improve with time and with specific exercises that help to strengthen the abdominal muscles. Surgery is rarely needed to treat diastasis recti. If you are concerned about the separation of your abdominal muscles, talk to your doctor or a qualified fitness professional.

Is diastasis recti serious?

A common concern for new mothers is diastasis recti, or separated abdominal muscles. This occurs when the connective tissue between the right and left sides of the rectus abdominis muscle stretches during pregnancy, making the abdomen appear wider. Diastasis recti is often accompanied by a bulge in the abdomen. Although it may be troubling to see this change in your body, diastasis recti is generally not a serious condition. There are a few things you can do to help heal diastasis recti. First, avoid any activity that puts strain on your abdominal muscles, such as sit-ups or crunches. Second, wear a supportive abdominal binder or girdle to help hold your muscles in place. Third, practice good posture and alignment. And finally, focus on strengthening your pelvic floor muscles. These muscles support your uterus, bladder, and rectum, and can help prevent incontinence, prolapse, and other issues. If you are still pregnant, there are some things you can do to help prevent diastasis recti. First, avoid gaining too much weight. Second, sleep on your side rather than on your back. Third, practice good posture and alignment. And fourth, do pelvic floor strengthening exercises. If you have diastasis recti, it is important to be patient. It can take several months for the connective tissue to heal and the muscles to come back together. With time and patience, you will see your belly go back to its pre-pregnancy state.

How can I fix diastasis recti naturally?

Since diastasis recti is a separation of the abdominal muscles, the first step is to bring those muscles back together. You can do this by doing planks and other exercises that work the transverse abdominis, the muscle that lies underneath the six-pack abs. Pilates is also beneficial. In addition to strengthening the muscles, you also need to work on your posture. Often, poor posture is the cause of diastasis recti. Strengthening the muscles can help, but it's also important to be aware of your posture and to correct it. Another important factor is your diet. Eating a diet that is high in processed foods and sugar can contribute to abdominal bloating and make the problem worse. Instead, focus on eating whole foods, like fruits, vegetables, and lean protein. Finally, it's important to be patient. Healing from diastasis recti takes time, so don't expect overnight results. Stick with it, and eventually, you will see improvement.

What exercises should I avoid with diastasis recti?

Exercises that put strain on the abdominal muscles, such as sit-ups and crunches, should be avoided with diastasis recti. Instead, opt for exercises that work the muscles around the abdomen, such as side-planks and Pilates. Overall, it is important to listen to your body and not push yourself too hard - back off from any exercises that cause pain or discomfort in the abdominal area. Pregnancy and diastasis recti can go hand-in-hand, unfortunately. The added strain on the abdominal muscles can cause the condition to worsen, or even develop in the first place. So, while you're expecting, be careful with your exercise routine and avoid anything that is too intense or puts too much strain on your stomach muscles. Once baby is born and you've been cleared by your doctor, you can begin slowly reintroducing more moderate exercises back into your life. In general, it's a good idea to focus on exercises that don't put a lot of strain on the abdominal muscles, such as walking, swimming, and riding a stationary bike. These activities will help you stay in shape without exacerbating your diastasis recti. As always, listen to your body and stop if you feel any pain or discomfort.

When is it too late to fix diastasis recti?

There's no definitive answer to this question - ultimately, it depends on the individual and the severity of their condition. However, as a general rule of thumb, it's usually best to seek treatment sooner rather than later. Diastasis recti is a condition where the abdominal muscles separate, causing a bulge in the stomach area. It's a relatively common issue, particularly among women who have recently given birth. The condition can cause a range of symptoms, from back pain and constipation, to bloating and a feeling of heaviness in the stomach area. If left untreated, diastasis recti can lead to more serious problems, such as hernias. In severe cases, surgery may be required to correct the problem. However, in most cases, diastasis recti can be treated with a combination of exercise and physiotherapy. The sooner you seek treatment for diastasis recti, the better. If you're unsure whether you have the condition, it's always best to speak to a doctor or physio. They will be able to assess your condition and advise you on the best course of treatment.

Diastasis recti is a separation of the abdominal muscles that can occur during pregnancy. The condition is often worsened by weight gain and may lead to back pain and other health problems. While there is no cure for diastasis recti, there are treatments that can help improve the condition.

Can you lose belly fat if you have diastasis recti?

Losing belly fat can be difficult, and it may seem impossible if you have diastasis recti. However, it is possible to lose belly fat, even with this condition. Diastasis recti is a condition where the abdominal muscles separate. This can happen during pregnancy, and it can also occur due to weight gain. The separated muscles can cause the belly to protrude. There are several things you can do to lose belly fat if you have diastasis recti. First, you need to focus on strengthening your core muscles. This can help to close the gap between your abdominal muscles and give you a flatter stomach. You can also try wearing a compression garment. This can help to hold your abdominal muscles in place and reduce the appearance of a bulging stomach. In addition, you need to make sure you are eating a healthy diet and getting enough exercise. Eating healthy foods will help you to lose weight, and exercise will help to tone your stomach muscles. If you are struggling to lose belly fat, you may want to talk to your doctor. They can provide you with guidance and support to help you reach your goals.

How do you get rid of belly fat with diastasis recti?

There are a few different ways that you can get rid of belly fat with diastasis recti. The first thing you need to do is to understand what diastasis recti is and how it affects your body. Diastasis recti is a condition where the abdominal muscles separate. This can occur during pregnancy, after a C-section, or even from weight gain. The separation of the muscles can cause the belly to protrude and look larger than it actually is. There are a few different exercises that you can do to help close the gap and get rid of the belly fat. One exercise is called the transverse abdominal crunch. This exercise helps to tone the muscles and close the gap. Another exercise is called the Pilates hundred. This exercise helps to strengthen the muscles and close the gap. You can also try wearing a compression garment. This will help to hold in the stomach and close the gap. There are a few different types of compression garments that you can choose from. You can wear a compression garment during the day and at night. If you are breastfeeding, you will want to make sure that you are doing Kegel exercises. These exercises help to tone the muscles that are used during breastfeeding. This can help to close the gap and get rid of the belly fat. You will also want to make sure that you are eating a healthy diet. Eating healthy foods will help to speed up the process of getting rid of the belly fat. You want to make sure that you are eating plenty of fruits, vegetables, and lean protein. You also want to make sure that you are drinking plenty of water. If you are not seeing results from these methods, you may want to consider surgery. Surgery is a last resort option for getting rid of the belly fat. There are a few different types of surgery that you can choose from. The type of surgery that you choose will depend on how severe your case is and how much fat you need to be removed. surgery is a last resort option for getting rid of the belly fat

What is the fastest way to fix diastasis recti?

A separation of the rectus abdominis muscle at the linea alba—commonly referred to as diastasis recti, or abdominal separation—is a condition that can occur during or after pregnancy. While the condition is more common in women who are pregnant (due to the added pressure on the abdominal muscles and connective tissue), it can also affect men and non-pregnant women. Diastasis recti is often diagnosed based on a physical examination, during which the width of the separation is measured. Once diagnosed, the condition can be treated with a variety of methods, including exercise, physical therapy, and surgery. While there is no one-size-fits-all answer to the question of how to fix diastasis recti, there are a few methods that are generally considered to be effective. One of the most important things you can do is to avoid exercises that put excessive pressure on the abdominal muscles, such as sit-ups and crunches. Instead, focus on exercises that strengthen the muscles without adding extra pressure, such as Pilates or yoga. There are also a number of specific exercises that can help to close the gap in the abdominal muscles, and these can be found in many online or print resources. In addition to exercise, wearing a supportive abdominal binder or garment can also help to minimize the appearance of diastasis recti and provide extra support to the muscles and connective tissue. If you are still pregnant, it is important to be aware of the risk of diastasis recti and to take steps to prevent it from happening. One of the best things you can do is to practice proper alignment and avoid positions that put pressure on the abdominal muscles, such as lying on your back with your legs in the air. Once your baby is born, be sure to take things slowly when it comes to resuming activity and avoid any forceful or repetitive motions that could exacerbate the condition. If you have diastasis recti and are not pregnant, you may be able to improve the condition with the help of a physical therapist. Physical therapists can teach you specific exercises and stretches to help close the gap in your abdominal muscles and improve your overall muscle tone. They can also give you guidance on how to modify your everyday activities to avoid making the condition worse. In some cases, surgery may be necessary to repair the abdominal muscles, but this is usually only recommended if other methods have been unsuccessful.

Is walking good for diastasis recti?

There is much debate in the medical community about whether or not walking is good for diastasis recti, a condition in which the abdominal muscles separate. Some doctors say that walking is fine, while others advise against it. The truth is that there is no definitive answer, as each case is different. Some people with diastasis recti find that walking aggravates their symptoms, while others find it helpful. If you have diastasis recti, you should listen to your body and do what feels right for you. If walking causes pain or makes your symptoms worse, you should stop doing it. However, if walking does not bother you, there is no reason to avoid it. Walking is a low-impact form of exercise, and it can be a good way to get some gentle activity if you are not able to do more strenuous exercise. If you are not sure whether or not walking is right for you, talk to your doctor. They will be able to give you more specific advice based on your individual case.

How long does it take to correct diastasis recti?

It is difficult to say how long it will take to correct diastasis recti as each individual is different. Some people may see improvement within a few weeks, while others may take longer. The key is to be consistent with your exercises and give your body time to heal. Diastasis recti is a separation of the abdominal muscles that often occurs during pregnancy. The condition can also occur in men and non-pregnant women, but it is most common in pregnant women. The condition is caused by the weakening of the connective tissue that holds the abdominal muscles together. The good news is that diastasis recti is fixable. The abdominal muscles can be strengthened and the connective tissue can be repaired. However, it will take time and consistency to see results. If you are pregnant and have diastasis recti, it is important to wait until after you have given birth to start exercises. Your body will need time to recover and heal. Once you have given birth, you can start slow with some basic exercises. The best exercises to strengthen the abdominal muscles are planks, Pilates, and sit-ups. Start with 1-2 sets of 10-15 repetitions and gradually increase as you get stronger. If you are not pregnant, you can start exercising right away. Again, start slow with 1-2 sets of 10-15 repetitions and gradually increase as you get stronger. Most importantly, be patient. It can take several weeks or months to see results. But if you are consistent with your exercises, you will eventually see a difference. If you have any pain or discomfort, please consult a medical professional.

What exercises fix diastasis recti?

There are a number of different exercises that can help to fix diastasis recti, and which ones will work best for you may depend on the severity of your condition. One exercise that can be effective is called the pelvic tilt. To do this, lie on your back with your knees bent and your feet flat on the ground. Slowly flatten your back against the floor and then tilt your pelvis upward, holding this position for a few seconds. Repeat this 10 times. Another exercise that can help is the double leg lift. This move targets the transverse abdominis, which is the deepest layer of abdominal muscles. To do it, lie on your back on the floor with your legs extended straight out in front of you and your arms at your sides. Slowly lift both legs off the ground, keeping them straight, and hold this position for a few seconds. Return to the starting position and repeat 10 times. If you have diastasis recti, it is also important to avoid any exercises that put unnecessary strain on your abdominal muscles, such as sit-ups or crunches. These can actually make the condition worse. Instead, focus on exercises that strengthen your overall core, such as Pilates or yoga.

Can you fix diastasis recti on your own?

There's no one-size-fits-all answer to this question - it depends on the individual case. The first step is to identify whether you have diastasis recti. This condition can be diagnosed by your GP, but there are also some simple tests you can do at home. Once you've established that you have diastasis recti, the next question is whether you can treat it yourself, or whether you need to seek professional help. If your case is mild, it's possible that you can improve the condition with some simple exercises and changes to your lifestyle. For example, you might need to avoid lifting heavy objects, or do some specific exercises to strengthening your abdominal muscles. However, if your diastasis recti is more severe, you'll probably need to see a physiotherapist or other medical professional. They can assess your individual case and devise a treatment plan that's right for you. This might involve a combination of exercises, massage, and other therapies. There's no quick fix for diastasis recti, and it can take some time to improve the condition. However, with the right treatment plan, it is possible to improve the symptoms and make a full recovery.

Diastasis recti is a condition in which the abdominal muscles separate. This can happen during pregnancy, but it can also occur without pregnancy. Diastasis recti can cause pain and difficulty with urination, constipation, and bloating. If you have diastasis recti, you may need to see a doctor to get treatment.

How do you close a diastasis recti gap?

A diastasis recti gap is a separation of the abdominal muscles. The gap can be caused by pregnancy, obesity, or other factors. To close a diastasis recti gap, the individual must first strengthen the muscles around the gap. This can be done through exercises that target the abdominal muscles, such as sit-ups, crunches, and planks. Once the muscles are strengthened, the individual can then begin to close the gap. There are a few ways to close the gap. One way is to do a surgery called an abdominoplasty, which involves making an incision in the lower abdomen and stitching the muscles together. Another way is to use a device called a tensioner, which is placed over the gap and pulls the muscles together. Lastly, there is a surgery called a myectomy, which removes excess tissue from around the gap. Whichever method is used, it is important to remember that it will take time and patience to close the diastasis recti gap.

Do belly bands help diastasis recti?

There is a lot of debate surrounding the use of belly bands for diastasis recti, with some people claiming that they are helpful and others asserting that they are not. So, what is the truth? Do belly bands help diastasis recti or not? Some people claim that belly bands can help to close the gap between the rectus abdominis muscles, which is what diastasis recti is. This is because when the muscles are brought closer together, it can help to provide support and stability to the abdomen. Additionally, it can also help to improve posture and prevent further separation of the muscles. However, there is no scientific evidence to support these claims. In fact, most experts agree that there is no evidence that any type of support band, including belly bands, can help to close the gap between the rectus abdominis muscles. Additionally, some experts believe that wearing a support band can actually make diastasis recti worse. So, what is the verdict? Are belly bands helpful for diastasis recti or not? Based on the available evidence, it seems that belly bands are not effective for treating diastasis recti. If you are looking for a way to treat your diastasis recti, you may want to consider other options, such as exercises that target the abdominal muscles.

Why do I have a bulge in the middle of my stomach when I do sit ups?

When you do a sit up, you're contracting your abs and trying to bring your rib cage closer to your pelvis. This works the abdominal muscles on the front and sides of your body, but it puts extra pressure on the connective tissue that runs down the center of your abs, called the linea alba. This pressure can cause the linea alba to stretch and thin out, eventually leading to a condition called diastasis recti. Diastasis recti can cause a bulge in your stomach, especially when you do sit ups. So why does this happen? Well, the linea alba is made up of collagen fibers, and like all connective tissue, itWeak connective tissue can be caused by a number of things, including: pregnancy obesity repeated strain on the abdominal muscles (from things like sit ups) Diastasis recti is more common in women who are pregnant or obese, but it can happen to anyone. If you're concerned that you may have diastasis recti, talk to your doctor. They can help you figure out if you have it and what you can do to treat it.

Can I do squats with diastasis recti?

diastasis recti, also known as abdominal distention, is a condition that can often be improved with physical activity and specific exercises. While the condition may make some activities, like squats, more difficult, they are not impossible to do. In fact, squats can actually help improve diastasis recti. Before beginning any sort of physical activity, it's important to check with a doctor, especially if you're pregnant or have any other health conditions. Once you get the okay from a medical professional, you can start slowly with bodyweight squats. Proper form is key when doing any type of squat, but it's especially important when you have diastasis recti. Start by standing with your feet shoulder-width apart. Slowly lower yourself down into a squatting position, keeping your back straight and your core engaged.

Once your thighs are parallel to the ground, slowly stand back up. You can also try adding a resistance band around your thighs for an extra challenge. If you're regularly doing bodyweight squats and are looking for a greater challenge, you can try adding weights. Start by holding a weight in each hand at arm's length. Keep your core engaged and slowly lower yourself into a squat. When your thighs are parallel to the ground, slowly stand back up. You can also try doing squat exercises with a barbell. Start by resting the barbell on your shoulders, making sure to keep your core engaged. Slowly lower yourself into a squatting position and then stand back up. While doing any type of squat will help strengthen your muscles and improve diastasis recti, it's important to remember to listen to your body. If you start to experience any pain, stop immediately and consult a doctor. With proper form and intensity, squats can be a great exercise for those with diastasis recti.

Is weight lifting good for diastasis recti?

If you have diastasis recti, weightlifting may help you heal. According to a study published in the journal BMC Women's Health, weightlifting can help improve the condition. The study looked at a group of women with diastasis recti who did weightlifting exercises three times a week for 12 weeks. The women who participated in the study saw a significant decrease in the separation of their rectus abdominis muscle, as well as an increase in muscle strength. In addition to weightlifting, the women in the study also performed exercises to improve their posture and abdominal muscle function. The results of the study suggest that a combination of weightlifting and other exercises may be the most effective approach to healing diastasis recti. If you're interested in trying weightlifting to heal your diastasis recti, it's important to consult with a doctor or physical therapist first. They can help you create a safe and effective workout plan.

How do you prevent diastasis recti from getting worse?

There isn't a one size fits all answer to preventing diastasis recti from worsening, as each individual case is unique. However, there are some general principles that can help. Firstly, it is important to avoid any activities or exercises that may put unnecessary strain on the abdominal muscles, such as sit-ups or crunches. If you are unsure whether an activity is safe, it is always best to consult with a medical professional. Secondly, it is important to strengthen the muscles around the abdomen, especially the transverse abdominis. This can be done through specific exercises, or simply by holding oneself in good posture throughout the day. Finally, it is essential to listen to your body and be aware of any changes that occur. If you notice any pain or discomfort, make sure to consult with a medical professional as soon as possible. By following these general principles, you can help prevent diastasis recti from worsening.

Is diastasis recti a hernia?

There is some confusion about whether or not diastasis recti is a hernia. In order to understand this, it is important to know what diastasis recti is and what hernias are. Diastasis recti is a separation of the abdominal muscles at the midline of the body. The muscles that are affected are the rectus abdominis, which are the large muscles that run down the front of the abdomen. These muscles are important in keeping the abdominal contents in place and helping with movements of the trunk. A hernia occurs when an organ or tissue protrudes through a weak spot in the muscle or surrounding tissue. Hernias can occur in different parts of the body, but are most common in the abdomen. The most common type of abdominal hernia is inguinal hernia, which is when a portion of the intestine protrudes through a weak spot in the groin. Hernias can also occur in the diaphragm, which is the muscle that separates the chest from the abdomen. So, diastasis recti is a separation of the abdominal muscles, while a hernia is a protrusion of an organ or tissue through a weak spot. Diastasis recti itself is not a hernia, but it can increase the risk of developing a hernia. This is because the separation of the muscles can create a weak spot in the abdominal wall. If there is increased pressure on the abdomen, such as during pregnancy or weightlifting, this can cause the organ or tissue to protrude through the weak spot. Diastasis recti is a common condition, especially after pregnancy. It is important to see a doctor if you are experiencing symptoms of diastasis recti, such as a bulge in the abdomen, abdominal pain, or difficulty moving the bowels. If you have diastasis recti, there are steps that you can take to help prevent a hernia from developing, such as avoiding heavy lifting and constipation.

Diastasis recti is a condition that can be caused by pregnancy, obesity, or other factors. It results in separation of the abdominal muscles, which can lead to back pain and other problems. Treatment involves exercises that help to strengthen the abdominal muscles.

Is diastasis recti surgery worth it?

The decision to have surgery is a personal one that depends on many factors. Some people may find that diastasis recti surgery improves their quality of life, while others may not feel that the benefits outweigh the risks. Here we will explore some of the key considerations that may help you decide whether or not diastasis recti surgery is right for you. Before considering surgery, it is important to speak with your doctor about all of the potential risks and benefits. Surgery is not without risks, and it is important to be sure that you are fully informed before making a decision. In addition to risks such as infection and bleeding, there is also the potential for complications such as seroma formation, which is the accumulation of fluid under the skin. Another important consideration is the cost of surgery. Diastasis recti surgery is not typically covered by insurance, so you will likely be responsible for the entire cost yourself. The cost can range from $3,000 to $10,000, depending on the extent of the surgery and the location where you have it done. Finally, you will need to consider the amount of time you are willing to take off from work or other activities to recover from surgery. The recovery process can vary from person to person, but you can expect to take at least a few weeks off to recover. After taking all of these factors into consideration, you can weigh the pros and cons of diastasis recti surgery to decide if it is right for you. If you do decide to have surgery, be sure to choose a board-certified plastic surgeon who has experience performing this type of procedure.

What does diastasis recti pain feel like?

When someone has diastasis recti, they may experience pain in the abdomen region. The pain can vary from person to person, but it is often described as a burning or aching sensation. Some people may only feel pain when they press on the affected area, while others may feel pain all the time. The pain may be worse when the person coughs, sneezes, or laughs. Diastasis recti can also cause difficulty urinating, as the urine may pass through the opening in the abdomen instead of through the urethra. In severe cases, hernias can develop, which can cause even more pain.

How to tell the difference between belly fat and diastasis recti?

There are a few key ways to tell the difference between belly fat and diastasis recti. First, check to see if your abdominal muscles have separated at the midline. This can be done by gently pressing your fingers into your stomach - if you can feel a gap between the muscles, it's likely you have diastasis recti. Another way to tell the difference is by observing how your stomach looks when you're standing up. People with diastasis recti will often have a 'pooch' or protrusion in the middle of their stomach, even when they're not overweight. This is caused by the separation of the abdominal muscles, which allows the internal organs to push through. Finally, you may also experience back pain and/or urinary incontinence if you have diastasis recti. This is because the separation of the abdominal muscles can put strain on the surrounding tissues and structures. If you're unsure whether you have belly fat or diastasis recti, it's best to see a doctor or certified personal trainer for a diagnosis. They will be able to confirm the diagnosis and advise you on the best course of treatment.

Does diastasis recti cause belly pooch?

A common worry among expectant mothers is that they will end up with a pooch after pregnancy, but what many don't realize is that diastasis recti—a condition where the abdominal muscles separate—is a leading cause of this. The good news is that there are things you can do to avoid it. Your abdominal muscles are key in supporting your back and keeping your spine in alignment. They also help you bend and twist. When they separate, it can cause a host of problems, including a noticeable bulge in your stomach, back pain, and difficulty moving. There are a number of things that can contribute to the development of diastasis recti, but the most common is pregnancy. The growing uterus puts pressure on the abdominal muscles, causing them to stretch and separate. This is why the condition is more common in women who have had multiple pregnancies. Other risk factors include being overweight or obese, carrying twins or multiples, and having a large baby. There is also a genetic component, so if your mother or grandmother had diastasis recti, you may be more likely to develop it yourself. The good news is that there are things you can do to prevent or minimize the risk of developing diastasis recti. First, avoid any activities that put unnecessary pressure on your abdomen, such as sit-ups, double leg lifts, and crunches. Second, focus on exercises that strengthen your deep abdominal muscles, such as Pilates or yoga. These exercises can help support your back and improve your posture, which can minimize the chances of your abdominal muscles separating. Finally, be sure to maintain a healthy weight. Gaining too much weight during pregnancy can put additional strain on your abdominal muscles and increase your risk of developing diastasis recti. If you do end up with diastasis recti, there are a number of treatments that can help, including physical therapy and surgery. In most cases, however, the condition will improve on its own over time. So, if you're concerned about developing a belly pooch after pregnancy, focus on preventing diastasis recti. By taking some simple precautions, you can help avoid this common condition and enjoy a happy, healthy postpartum recovery.

What exercise makes diastasis recti worse?

When it comes to exercise and diastasis recti, there are certain movements that can make the condition worse. These exercises put unnecessary strain on the abdominal muscles and can cause the rectus abdominis muscle to separate further. Some of the exercises that can make diastasis recti worse include crunches, sit-ups, and any activity that involves twisting or flexing of the torso. These movements put additional pressure on the abdominal muscles and can cause the rectus abdominis to separate further. Additionally, any exercise that increases intra-abdominal pressure can also worsen diastasis recti. This includes activities like heavy lifting, powerlifting, and Olympic weightlifting. These activities place strain on the abdominal muscles and can cause the rectus abdominis to separate further. If you have diastasis recti, it's important to avoid these exercises and movements that can make the condition worse. Instead, focus on exercises that don't put unnecessary strain on the abdominal muscles. These exercises can help you strengthen your core without making your diastasis recti worse.

Does diastasis recti make me look pregnant?

Symptoms of diastasis recti can closely resemble those of pregnancy, including a protruding abdomen. This can lead some to wonder if diastasis recti makes them look pregnant. While a protruding abdomen is a common symptom of diastasis recti, it is not the only symptom. Diastasis recti can also cause back pain and difficulty completing everyday activities, such as bending down or coughing. Diastasis recti is a condition that results from the separation of the abdominal muscles. This separation can occur during pregnancy, but it can also occur in both men and women who are not pregnant. Diastasis recti is a relatively common condition, affecting about 33% of pregnant women. If you are concerned that you may have diastasis recti, it is important to speak with a doctor. They will be able to confirm the diagnosis and develop a treatment plan. Treatment for diastasis recti may include exercises to help improve muscle function and strength, as well as weight loss if needed. Surgery is also an option for some people with diastasis recti. While diastasis recti can cause a person to appear pregnant, it is important to remember that it is a separate condition with its own set of symptoms. If you are experiencing symptoms of diastasis recti, speak with a doctor to develop a treatment plan that is right for you.

Does diastasis recti cause bloating?

Most people think of bloating as something that happens when you eat too much. But for some people, bloating is a chronic condition that can be extremely painful. And for some people with bloating, the cause is diastasis recti. Diastasis recti is a condition that occurs when the abdominal muscles separate. This separation can cause the belly to protrude and look bloated. Diastasis recti is common after pregnancy, but it can also occur in men and women who are not pregnant. So, does diastasis recti cause bloating? The answer is yes, diastasis recti can cause bloating. But not everyone with diastasis recti will experience bloating. And not everyone with bloating has diastasis recti. There are many possible causes of bloating, including food intolerance, constipation, irritable bowel syndrome, and certain medications. But if you have chronic bloating and you also have diastasis recti, there's a good chance that the two conditions are connected. If you suspect that you have diastasis recti, talk to your doctor. They can perform a physical exam and order tests to confirm the diagnosis. If you do have diastasis recti, there are treatments that can help. These include exercises to improve muscle tone and strength, and surgery to repair the abdominal muscles. If you have diastasis recti and you're struggling with bloating, know that you're not alone. There are many people in the same boat. But there are also treatments that can help. So talk to your doctor and find a treatment plan that works for you.

Diastasis recti, or abdominal separation, is a condition that can occur during pregnancy when the abdominal muscles separate. This can cause a bulge in the belly and may make it difficult to do certain activities, such as sit-ups. A weak core can also lead to back pain. There is no cure for diastasis recti, but there are things that can be done to help improve the condition, such as exercises that strengthen the abdominal muscles.

Does physio help diastasis recti?

It is not uncommon for women to experience abdominal separation, or diastasis recti, during pregnancy. The condition occurs when the abdominal muscles widen and the connective tissue between them stretches. This can cause the abdomen to protrude and can lead to back pain and other issues. While there is no cure for diastasis recti, there are treatments that can help improve the condition. One such treatment is physical therapy. Physical therapy can help to strengthen the muscles and connective tissue around the abdomen, which can help to improve the appearance of the abdomen and reduce pain. There is no guarantee that physical therapy will help every case of diastasis recti, but it is often worth trying if other treatments have not been successful. If you are considering physical therapy, be sure to consult with a qualified physical therapist to ensure that you are getting the best possible care.

Why does diastasis recti happen?

It's not entirely clear what causes diastasis recti, but there are some theories. One is that it's due to pregnancy and childbirth. The abdominal muscles are stretched during pregnancy, and they don't always snap back into place after the baby is born. childbirth. Another possibility is that diastasis recti is genetic. If your parents or grandparents had it, you may be more likely to have it, too. It's also possible that being overweight or obese increases your risk of developing diastasis recti. That's because carrying extra weight puts additional strain on your abdominal muscles. If you have diastasis recti, you may be wondering how to fix it. Unfortunately, there's no guaranteed way to get rid of the condition. If it's mild, you may be able to improve it with exercise and physical therapy. If it's more severe, you may need surgery. If you're considering surgery, it's important to talk to a experienced surgeon. They can help you weigh the risks and benefits, and decide if surgery is the right choice for you.

What are the symptoms of abdominal separation?

When the abdominal muscles separate, it is called abdominal separation, or diastasis recti. The main symptom is a bulge in the middle of the abdomen, caused by the separation of the rectus abdominis muscle. This bulge may be more noticeable when lying down, and may cause pain or Difficulty when moving. Other symptoms may include urinary incontinence, constipation, and hernias. Most cases of abdominal separation are caused by pregnancy, but it can also be caused by obesity, chronic cough, and other conditions. Treatment typically involves physical therapy and exercises to strengthen the abdominal muscles. Surgery is generally only recommended if the abdominal separation is severe and causing significant pain or other problems.

How long does it take to fix abdominal separation?

Abdominal separation, or diastasis recti, is a condition that can occur during or after pregnancy. The abdominal muscles stretch and separate, normally coming back together after the baby is born. However, in some cases the separation does not heal properly and the stomach bulges out. This can cause back pain and make it difficult to do everyday activities. So how long does it take to fix abdominal separation? Unfortunately, there is no easy answer. It depends on the severity of the separation, how long ago it occurred, and whether you are doing any exercises or physical therapy to help heal the separation. If the separation is mild, it may heal on its own within a few months. However, if the separation is more severe, it may take up to a year or longer to heal. There are a few things you can do to help heal abdominal separation. First, you can try exercises that help strengthen the abdominal muscles. These may include crunches, sit-ups, and leg raises. You can also try wearing a support belt to help hold the stomach in place. If you are still having pain or difficulty after trying these things, you may need to see a doctor or physical therapist. They can help you come up with a more specific plan to help heal your abdominal separation. It is important to remember that healing times vary from person to person. Some people may heal quickly, while others may take longer. If you are concerned about your healing time, be sure to talk to your doctor.

Will diastasis recti heal on its own?

When it comes to diastasis recti, or a separation of the abdominal muscles, many people want to know if it will heal on its own. The answer to this question is both yes and no. In some cases, diastasis recti will heal without intervention, while in other cases, it may require surgery to correct the problem. The severity of diastasis recti will play a role in whether or not it will heal on its own. In mild cases, the rectus abdominis, or abdominal muscles, will gradually begin to heal on their own. This is usually a slow process, however, and can take several months. In more severe cases, the muscles may not heal properly on their own, and surgery may be required to correct the problem. One of the main reasons diastasis recti may not heal on its own is due to the repeated strain that is placed on the abdominal muscles. Every time you cough, sneeze, laugh, or bear down, you are placing strain on your abdominal muscles. This strain can cause the muscles to separate even further, and can make it difficult for them to heal properly. If you are hoping to avoid surgery, there are some things you can do to help the healing process. First, it is important to avoid any activities that place strain on the abdominal muscles. This includes coughing, sneezing, laughing, and bearing down. Second, you can do abdominal exercises that help to strengthen the muscles and promote healing. Finally, you can wear a supportive garment, such as a belt or binder, to help hold the muscles in place and prevent further separation. If you have diastasis recti, it is important to talk to your doctor about the best treatment option for you. In some cases, surgery may be the best option, while in others, conservative treatment may be all that is needed. No matter what route you decide to go, however, it is important to get treatment as soon as possible to promote healing and avoid further complications.

How do you fix abdominal separation?

Having a baby is an amazing time full of new experiences, but it can also take a toll on your body – especially your abdominal muscles. The added weight of pregnancy and nursing can cause the abdominal muscles to separate, a condition known as diastasis recti or abdominal separation. How do you know if you have diastasis recti? There are a few tell-tale signs of abdominal separation. First, you may notice a bulge in your abdomen, especially when you strain or contract your abdominal muscles. You may also feel a separation between your abdominal muscles when you press on your stomach. Finally, you may notice that your belly button sticks out more than usual. If you suspect you have diastasis recti, you can check by lying down on your back with your knees bent. Place your fingers just above your belly button and press gently. If you can feel a gap of more than 2.5 cm (1 inch), you likely have abdominal separation. What causes abdominal separation? Abdominal separation is caused by the added pressure on the abdominal muscles during pregnancy. The extra weight of the baby and the amniotic fluid stretches the connective tissue that holds the abdominal muscles together. For some women, the connective tissue may not completely return to its original strength and position after pregnancy, resulting in abdominal separation. How can you fix abdominal separation? There are a few things you can do to help heal abdominal separation. First, you should avoid any activities that put strain on your abdominal muscles, such as sit-ups, double leg lifts, and crunching movements. Instead, focus on exercises that strengthen the deep abdominal muscles, such as Pilates or yoga. You can also help heal abdominal separation by wearing a supportive band or wrap. These can help hold the abdominal muscles in place and take some of the pressure off of the connective tissue. Finally, give your body time to heal. Abdominal separation is a common condition and usually gets better on its own within a few months. However, if you have severe abdominal separation, you may need to see a physical therapist or doctor for help.

What does your stomach look like if you have diastasis recti?

When you have diastasis recti, your stomach muscles become separated at the midline. This can cause your stomach to protrude outwards and may make you look pregnant, even if you're not. The separation of your muscles can also cause back pain and make it difficult to do certain exercises, such as sit-ups. In severe cases, diastasis recti can lead to hernias. If you have diastasis recti, you may notice that your stomach bulges out when you sit up or stand. The separation of your abdominal muscles can also cause your stomach to protrude when you're lying down. In some cases, the protrusion may be severe enough that it's visible through your clothes. If you have diastasis recti, you may notice that your stomach feels soft and mushy. This is because the separation of your muscles allows your internal organs to press against your abdominal wall. In severe cases, the protrusion of your stomach may make it difficult to breathe. If you think you may have diastasis recti, it's important to see a doctor. They can confirm the diagnosis with a physical examination and order additional tests, if needed. Treatment for diastasis recti usually focuses on improving the strength and function of the abdominal muscles. This can be done through physical therapy, exercises, and splinting. In some cases, surgery may be necessary to correct the condition.

Diastasis recti is a condition in which the stomach muscles separate at the midline. This condition is common in pregnant women and can lead to back pain and hernias. Diastasis recti can be corrected with surgery.

Does diastasis recti cause big belly?

Many women seek ways to slim down their bodies, particularly after having children. One common concern among mothers is whether diastasis recti, a condition involving the separation of abdominal muscles, causes a big belly. While it's true that diastasis recti can cause a noticeable protrusion in the abdomen, there are ways to manage the condition and avoid letting it impact your body confidence. Diastasis recti occurs when the rectus abdominis muscles, which run down the center of the stomach, separate at the midline. This can cause the stomach to protrude, particularly in the lower abdomen. The condition is common among pregnant women and women who have recently given birth. It's also more likely to occur in women who are overweight or have had multiple pregnancies. While diastasis recti can cause a noticeable bulge in the stomach, it doesn't necessarily mean that you have a big belly. There are a number of factors that can contribute to abdominal size, including excess weight, bloating, and water retention. If you're concerned about the way your stomach looks, it's best to talk to your doctor. They can help you determine whether diastasis recti is the cause of your concerns and advise you on the best way to manage the condition. There are a number of ways to treat diastasis recti, including exercises that can help to close the gap between the abdominal muscles. Surgery is also an option, but it's typically only recommended for severe cases. If you're looking to avoid surgery, there are a number of devices, such as abdominal binders, that can help to support the stomach and give the appearance of a slimmer waistline. While diastasis recti can be a cause of concern for many women, it's important to remember that there are ways to manage the condition. With the right treatment, you can avoid letting diastasis recti impact your body confidence.

What makes diastasis recti worse?

There are many things that can contribute to making diastasis recti worse. First and foremost, if you are pregnant, continuing to gain weight can put undue stress on your abdominal muscles and make the diastasis recti worse. Additionally, anything that increases intra-abdominal pressure can also worsen diastasis recti. This includes things like coughing, sneezing, laughing, constipation, and even holding your breath. Additionally, improper form during exercises can also worsen diastasis recti. So, if you are already dealing with this condition, it is important to be mindful of how you are working out. For instance, doing crunches or sit-ups can actually put more strain on your abdominal muscles and make the diastasis recti worse. The same goes for lifting weights—you want to be careful not to overdo it and put unnecessary strain on your abdominal muscles. Lastly, we know that is it is possible for diastasis recti to run in families, so if you have a family history of the condition, you may be more likely to develop it or to have it worsen. If you are pregnant and have diastasis recti, or if you are concerned that you may be developing the condition, it is important to speak with your doctor. They can give you specific guidance on how to care for your condition and help you avoid things that may make it worse.

Can diastasis recti open again?

As your stomach or abdomen grows during pregnancy, the connective tissue between your rectus abdominis muscles stretches. This condition is called diastasis recti or DR. DR happens when the connective tissue stretches too much and becomes thin. The rectus abdominis muscles are the long muscles that go down the center of your stomach. They're also known as the "six-pack" muscles. After you give birth, the muscles and connective tissue often return to their original state. But in some cases, the DR might not improve on its own. Whether or not you have DR, you can do things to help improve the muscle separation. If you have DR, you might be wondering, "Can diastasis recti open again?" The answer is yes, but it's not very common. If you have DR and you get pregnant again, it's possible that the DR could open up again. But it's not likely to happen if you don't have DR. If you have DR and you want to prevent it from opening up again, there are some things you can do. First, you can try to avoid gaining too much weight during pregnancy. You can also do some pelvic floor muscle exercises and abdominal exercises to help improve your muscle tone. And lastly, you can wear a belly support band or girdle to help hold your muscles and connective tissue in place. If you're pregnant and you have DR, talk to your doctor about ways to prevent it from opening up again. And if you're thinking about getting pregnant again, talk to your doctor about your risk for DR.

How can I flatten my diastasis recti?

A lot of people have asked me how they can flatten their diastasis recti, so I wrote this little guide on the subject. I hope it will be of some help! First and foremost, diastasis recti is not something that can be fixed with surgery. So, if you're looking for a quick fix, you're out of luck. That being said, there are a few things you can do to help improve the appearance of your diastasis recti. First, make sure you're doing regular core exercises. This will help to strengthen the muscles around your stomach, which can help to pull in your stomach and make your diastasis recti less visible. Second, try wearing a compression garment. This can help to hold in your stomach and give the appearance of a flatter stomach. Finally, make sure you're staying hydrated. Drinking plenty of water will help to keep your skin looking healthy and can help to reduce the appearance of wrinkles and fine lines. So, there you have it! A few tips on how you can improve the appearance of your diastasis recti. Remember, there is no quick fix, but with a little effort, you can see a noticeable difference.

What exercise closes diastasis recti?

There is no single exercise that will definitively close diastasis recti, but there are certain exercises that can help. One effective way to help close the gap is to exercise the abdominal muscles. This can be done through crunches, sit-ups, and other exercises that target the abs. Additionally, exercises that strengthen the muscles around the abdominal area can also help to close the gap. These include exercises like leg raises and planks. While there is no guarantee that any exercise will close diastasis recti, these exercises can help to improve the condition. Additionally, it is important to seek professional help if the condition is severe. This is because diastasis recti can sometimes lead to hernias. If you suspect that you have diastasis recti, it is important to speak to a doctor or other healthcare professional.

Is abdominal separation painful?

Most new mothers are surprised to discover that abdominal separation is a common postpartum condition. Many are also surprised to learn that it can be quite painful. Abdominal separation, also known as diastasis recti, is a condition that can occur when the muscles of the abdomen are stretched and damaged during pregnancy. This can cause the muscles to separate at the center of the abdomen. While abdominal separation is not dangerous, it can cause a great deal of pain. Many women report feeling a sharp pain in their abdomen when they cough, sneeze, or laugh. Others find that simple movements, such as getting out of bed or standing up from a chair, can be extremely painful. There are several things that can be done to help ease the pain of abdominal separation. First, it is important to avoid any activities that put strain on the abdominal muscles, such as lifting heavy objects or doing sit-ups. Second, wearing a supportive abdominal binder can help to take some of the pressure off of the muscles. Finally,massaging the muscles of the abdomen can also help to reduce pain and inflammation. If you are dealing with the pain of abdominal separation, it is important to talk to your doctor. They can help you find ways to ease your pain and avoid further damage to your abdominal muscles.

How long does it take to heal diastasis recti with exercise?

How long does it take to heal diastasis recti with exercise? It is estimated that diastasis recti affects 33% of women. Diastasis recti is a condition where the abdominal muscles separate, and can be caused by pregnancy, obesity, and age. The condition can be healed with exercise, but it is important to note that it may take some time to see results. One study found that it took 16 weeks of targeted exercise to significantly improve the condition in a group of women with diastasis recti. The women in the study exercised for 30 minutes, five times per week. They focused on exercises that engaged the transverse abdominal muscles, which are the muscles that run along the sides of the body and help to stabilize the spine. While it may take some time to heal diastasis recti with exercise, it is an effective treatment option for many women. If you are interested in trying exercise to improve your condition, be sure to speak with your doctor first. They can help you to develop a safe and effective exercise plan that is tailored to your specific needs.

The condition known as diastasis recti is a separation of the abdominal muscles that can occur during pregnancy. It is a common condition, and usually resolves itself after pregnancy. However, in some cases, the separation does not heal properly and can cause ongoing problems. Diastasis recti can cause weakening of the abdominal muscles and back pain. It can also make it difficult to lose weight after pregnancy. If you are suffering from diastasis recti, there are treatments available that can help.

When should I worry about diastasis recti?

When it comes to diastasis recti, there are a few general guidelines to follow. If you have a noticeable bulge in your abdomen, especially when lying down or bending over, this is cause for concern. Additionally, if you feel pain or discomfort in your abdomen, especially when coughing or sneezing, this may also indicate that you have diastasis recti. Of course, it is always best to consult with a medical professional if you have any concerns about diastasis recti. They will be able to give you a more specific answer based on your individual circumstances. However, in general, if you are experiencing any of the symptoms mentioned above, it is important to seek medical attention. Left untreated, diastasis recti can lead to a number of complications, such as hernias, incontinence, and chronic low back pain. Therefore, it is important to be vigilant about any changes or problems you are experiencing in your abdomen. If you have any concerns, be sure to speak to a doctor as soon as possible.

How can I prevent diastasis recti from getting worse?

Diastasis recti is a condition in which the stomach muscles stretch and separate. This can cause the stomach to protrude and the back to arch. Diastasis recti is common during pregnancy, but can also occur after pregnancy, due to weight gain or other factors. There are several things you can do to prevent diastasis recti from getting worse. First, avoid activities that put unnecessary strain on your stomach muscles, such as sit-ups, crunches, and other abdominal exercises. Second, maintain a healthy weight. If you are overweight, losing weight can help reduce the strain on your stomach muscles and improve your overall health. Third, eat a healthy diet. Eating a diet rich in fruits, vegetables, and whole grains can help support your body and reduce the risk of diastasis recti. fourth, practice good posture. Slouching puts additional strain on your stomach muscles, so practice sitting and standing up straight. Finally, wear supportive clothing. Wearing a supportive belt or garment can help prevent the stomach from protruding and putting strain on the muscles. By following these simple tips, you can prevent diastasis recti from getting worse and improve your overall health.

Will losing weight get rid of diastasis?

New studies suggest that diastasis recti, otherwise known as abdominal separation, is more common than previously thought. This condition occurs when the connective tissue between the left and right sides of the rectus abdominis muscle—the so-called "six-pack" muscle—stretches or tears. This can happen during pregnancy as the abdominal muscles adjust to accommodate the growing uterus, but it can also occur in non-pregnant adults due to factors such as chronic cough, obesity, and even regular sit-ups and crunches. So, what does this mean if you have diastasis recti and you're hoping to lose weight? Unfortunately, there's no easy answer. Losing weight may help to improve the appearance of diastasis recti, but it won't necessarily get rid of the condition. This is because the damage to the connective tissue is often permanent. Even if you lose a significant amount of weight, you may still have some looseness in your abdominal muscles. That said, losing weight can still be beneficial for people with diastasis recti. In addition to helping improve the appearance of the condition, it can also help to lessen the risk of other health problems that are associated with obesity, such as heart disease, type 2 diabetes, and certain types of cancer. So, while losing weight may not get rid of diastasis recti completely, it can still be a helpful step to take.

Can a waist trainer fix diastasis recti?

There's no one-size-fits-all answer to this question - it depends on the severity of your diastasis recti, and how committed you are to wearing a waist trainer. That said, a study published in the International Journal of Sports Physical Therapy in 2016 found that wearing a compression garment (like a waist trainer) can help with diastasis recti, providing you also do exercises to strengthen your core muscles. So, if you have mild diastasis recti and you're willing to wear a waist trainer regularly, it's possible that it could help fix the problem. However, if your diastasis recti is more severe, it's unlikely that a waist trainer will be enough on its own - you'll need to see a doctor or physiotherapist for advice on exercises and other treatments.

What foods should I avoid with diastasis recti?

There are a few types of foods that you should avoid if you have diastasis recti. These include: 1) Foods that are high in sugar. This includes things like candy, cake, cookies, and other sweets. Too much sugar can worsen inflammation and make it harder for your body to heal. 2) Foods that are high in saturated fat. This includes things like fatty cuts of meat, full-fat dairy products, and processed foods. Too much saturated fat can lead to weight gain, which can further worsen diastasis recti. 3) Foods that are high in salt. This includes things like chips, pretzels, and other salty snacks. Too much salt can cause bloating and water retention, which can make diastasis recti worse. 4) Alcohol. Alcohol can cause dehydration and inflammation, both of which can make diastasis recti worse. 5) caffeine. Caffeine can cause dehydration and also interfere with sleep, both of which can worsen diastasis recti. In general, it's best to eat a healthy diet that includes plenty of fruits, vegetables, and whole grains. Avoiding processed foods, sugary drinks, and excessive amounts of saturated fat, salt, and caffeine will help you keep diastasis recti under control.

Are squats OK for diastasis recti?

If you have diastasis recti, you may be wondering if it's OK to do squats. The answer is that it depends. If your diastasis recti is severe, then you shouldn't do squats. However, if your diastasis recti is mild, then you can try doing squats with light weights. Diastasis recti is a condition where the abdominal muscles separate. This can happen during pregnancy, but it can also happen to anyone, even if they've never been pregnant. Diastasis recti can cause pain and weakness in the abdominal muscles. If you have diastasis recti, you should avoid doing any exercises that put strain on the abdominal muscles, like sit-ups, crunches, and leg lifts. These exercises can make the diastasis recti worse. Squats are an exercise that put strain on the abdominal muscles. However, if you have mild diastasis recti, you can try doing squats with light weights. If you start to feel pain, stop doing the squats. If you have diastasis recti, you should talk to your doctor before starting any exercise program. They can help you determine if squats are safe for you.

Does diastasis recti get worse with age?

As we age, our skin loses elasticity and our muscles weaken. Unfortunately, diastasis recti can worsen with age. The connective tissue between our abdominal muscles stretches and weakens, making it harder for our muscles to support our spine and internal organs. This can cause a number of problems, such as back pain, digestive issues, and urinary incontinence. While there is no cure for diastasis recti, there are certain things you can do to improve the condition. Exercises that target the abdominal muscles, such as crunches, can help to strengthen the muscles and improve support for the spine. Wearing a supportive belt or girdle can also help to improve the condition by providing additional support for the abdominal muscles. If you are concerned about the effects of diastasis recti, talk to your doctor. They can assess the severity of your condition and recommend the best course of treatment. In some cases, surgery may be recommended to Repair the stretched or torn connective tissue.

While diastasis recti is a common condition, it is often misunderstood. Many people think that it is a hernia, when in fact it is a separation of the abdominal muscles. Diastasis recti can occur in both men and women, but is more common in women who have had multiple pregnancies. The condition is usually benign and does not require treatment, but can lead to back pain and other problems if left untreated.

Will push ups worsen diastasis recti?

There is a lot of debate surrounding exercise and diastasis recti, with some people saying that certain exercises can make the condition worse. One exercise that is often cited as being particularly harmful is the push up. So, will doing push ups make diastasis recti worse? There is no definitive answer, as everyone is different and will react differently to exercise. However, there are a few things to bear in mind. Firstly, when doing any kind of exercise, it is important to listen to your body. If something hurts, then stop. With diastasis recti, there is a risk of further weakening the abdominal muscles, so it is important to be careful. Secondly, the way you do a push up can also make a difference. If you do them with poor form, then you are more likely to hurt yourself. Make sure you keep your back straight, and don't let your hips sag. Finally, if you are pregnant or have recently had a baby, then you should avoid doing any kind of strenuous exercise. Your body is already under a lot of strain, and you don't want to risk making things worse. So, in conclusion, whether or not push ups will make diastasis recti worse is something that is individual to each person. However, it is important to be careful when exercising, and to listen to your body. If you are unsure, then it is always best to speak to a medical professional before starting any new exercise regime.

Can you live with diastasis recti?

The condition known as diastasis recti is characterized by a separation of the abdominal muscles along the midline of the stomach. This can happen during pregnancy, but it can also occur due to other causes, such as excess weight or age-related weakening of the muscles. The separation of the muscles can range from a tiny gap to a complete rupture, and the condition can lead to a number of different symptoms. Some people with diastasis recti may experience abdominal pain, hernias, or difficulty moving the bowels. Others may have no symptoms at all. Diastasis recti is not a life-threatening condition, and most people who have it can live relatively normal lives. However, the condition can be associated with some serious health problems, so it is important to seek medical attention if you think you may have it. In some cases, surgery may be necessary to repair the separated muscles. Even if surgery is not required, your doctor may recommend specific exercises and physical therapy to help you strengthen the muscles and minimize the symptoms. Living with diastasis recti can be challenging, but it is possible to manage the condition and live a normal, healthy life. If you are concerned that you may have diastasis recti, talk to your doctor. They can help you develop a treatment plan that is right for you.

How much does diastasis surgery cost?

When it comes to diastasis surgery, there is no one-size-fits-all answer when it comes to pricing. The cost of the surgery will vary depending on a number of factors, including the severity of the condition, the type of procedure being performed, the experience of the surgeon, and the geographical location. In general, however, patients can expect to pay somewhere in the range of $3,000 to $10,000 for diastasis surgery. While the cost of diastasis surgery may seem like a lot of money up front, it is important to keep in mind that this is a surgery that can potentially have a life-changing effect. For many patients, the surgery is able to correct a condition that has caused them a great deal of pain and discomfort for many years. In addition, the surgery can also help to improve the patient's appearance, which can boost their self-confidence. If you are considering diastasis surgery, it is important to consult with a board-certified plastic surgeon who has experience with this type of procedure. During your consultation, the surgeon will be able to evaluate your individual case and provide you with a more accurate estimate of the surgery's cost.

How much does it cost to repair diastasis?

The average cost of surgery to repair diastasis recti is between $3,000 and $6,000. This will usually cover the cost of the procedure itself, as well as any necessary anesthesia and post-operative care. However, it is important to keep in mind that this is just an average cost, and the actual price will vary depending on a number of factors, such as the surgeon's fee, the hospital's charges, and the patient's insurance coverage. There are a number of different techniques that can be used to repair diastasis recti, and the type of surgery that is best for a particular patient will depend on a number of factors, such as the severity of the condition, the patient's age and health, and the surgeon's preference. In some cases, the surgeon may opt for a less invasive approach, such as a procedure known as an abdominal plication, which can be done through laparoscopic surgery. In other cases, a more traditional approach, such as a tummy tuck, may be necessary. The cost of surgery to repair diastasis recti will also vary depending on the extent of the surgery that is required. In cases where only a small area is affected, the surgery may be fairly quick and straightforward. However, in cases where the condition is more severe, the surgery may be more complex and take longer to complete. In most cases, patients who undergo surgery to repair diastasis recti will need to stay in the hospital for one or two nights. However, in some cases, patients may be able to go home the same day. The length of the hospital stay will depend on the type of surgery that was performed and the patient's individual recovery. Most patients who have surgery to repair diastasis recti will be able to return to their normal activities within a few weeks. However, it is important to keep in mind that it may take several months for the incisions to heal completely. Additionally, patients may need to take it easy for the first few weeks, avoiding strenuous activity and lifting heavy objects.

How painful is diastasis recti surgery?

Diastasis recti, also known as abdominal separation, is a condition where the rectus abdominis muscles separate at the midline of the stomach. This condition is relatively common, especially among pregnant women and women who have recently given birth. Diastasis recti can cause a number of problems, including pain in the lower back and abdomen, hernias, and incontinence. Diastasis recti surgery is a relatively simple procedure that is typically performed as an outpatient procedure. The surgery involves stitching the muscles back together using a piece of surgical tape. The surgery itself is usually not painful, although there may be some discomfort afterwards as the muscles heal. Recovery from diastasis recti surgery is typically fairly quick, and most people are able to return to their normal activities within a few weeks.

What causes diastasis recti in females?

There are numerous factors that can contribute to the development of diastasis recti in females. Pregnancy is one of the most common causes, as the expanding uterus can put added pressure on the abdominal muscles and cause them to separate. Other causes can include obesity, chronic coughing or sneezing, and even certain types of exercise. Pregnancy is thought to be the most common cause of diastasis recti in females. As the uterus expands during pregnancy, it puts added pressure on the abdominal muscles. This can cause the muscles to separate, and in some cases, the separation may not heal completely after the baby is born. obesity can also contribute to diastasis recti, as the extra weight can put added pressure on the abdominal muscles. chronic coughing or sneezing can also cause the abdominal muscles to separate, as can certain types of exercise. If you are pregnant and think you may have diastasis recti, it is important to talk to your doctor. They can assess your abdominal muscles and determine if you have a separation. If you do have a separation, there are a few things you can do to help treat it. First, you can try to avoid activities that put added pressure on your abdominal muscles. This includes things like lifting heavy objects, coughing or sneezing forcefully, and doing sit-ups or crunches. You can also try to wear a supportive garment, like a belly band, to help hold your muscles in place. If your separation is severe, you may need to have surgery to repair it. Diastasis recti is a condition that can be caused by various factors, but is most commonly seen in pregnant women. The condition can cause the abdominal muscles to separate, and can sometimes lead to complications like hernias. If you think you may have diastasis recti, be sure to talk to your doctor so they can assess your condition and recommend the best course of treatment.

What is the cause of hanging belly?

The condition known as diastasis recti is caused by a separation of the abdominal muscles at the midline of the stomach. This can occur during pregnancy as the baby grows and puts pressure on the muscles, causing them to stretch and separate. The result is a stomach that protrudes outward and gives the appearance of a hanging belly. Often, post-pregnancy women seek surgical correction to repair the abdominal muscles. However, there are also some exercises that can help to improve the condition. The most common cause of diastasis recti is pregnancy. As the baby grows, it puts pressure on the abdominal muscles, causing them to stretch and separate. This can happen even in healthy pregnancies. In some cases, the separation may only be partial, while in others it can be complete. After the baby is born, the separation typically heals on its own. However, in some cases, the muscles may not heal properly, resulting in a condition known as diastasis recti. There are also other causes of diastasis recti, though they are less common. Obesity can cause the abdominal muscles to stretch and separate, as can repetitive movements such as sit-ups or crunches. Age can also play a role, as the abdominal muscles can begin to weaken with age, making them more susceptible to separation. The main symptom of diastasis recti is a protruding stomach. This can occur even in healthy pregnancies. However, it is more likely to occur in women who are obese or have had multiple pregnancies. Often, the protrusion is more noticeable after the baby is born. In some cases, the protrusion may be accompanied by back pain, as the separated abdominal muscles can put pressure on the lower back. Diastasis recti is typically diagnosed through a physical exam. The doctor will look for a separation of the abdominal muscles at the midline of the stomach. In some cases, an MRI or CT scan may be ordered to confirm the diagnosis. There is no single treatment for diastasis recti. In many cases, the condition will improve on its own over time. However, there are some exercises that can help to improve the condition. These exercises focus on strengthening the abdominal muscles and helping them to heal. In severe cases, surgery may be required to repair the abdominal muscles.

Diastasis recti, or abdominal separation, is a condition that can occur during pregnancy when the growing uterus stretches the abdominal muscles. This can cause a bulge in the abdomen and pain. Diastasis recti usually improves after pregnancy, but it can sometimes persist and may require surgery to correct.

What causes hanging belly after pregnancy?

After a pregnancy, many women are left with a hanging belly. This can be caused by a number of things, including weak abdominal muscles, excess weight, and fluid retention. Weak abdominal muscles are a common cause of a hanging belly after pregnancy. The abdominal muscles are stretched during pregnancy, and they may not return to their pre-pregnancy state. This can cause the belly to sag and look hanging. Excess weight can also cause a hanging belly after pregnancy. The extra weight can pull down on the skin and muscles, causing the belly to sag. diet and exercise can help to reduce the amount of excess weight, and help to tone the abdominal muscles. Fluid retention is another common cause of a hanging belly after pregnancy. The body retains extra fluid during pregnancy, and this can cause the belly to look swollen and hanging. Fluid retention usually goes away on its own, but it can be helped by wearing compression garments and by doing things to help reduce swelling, such as sleeping on your left side and elevating your feet when you can. There are a number of things that can cause a hanging belly after pregnancy. Weak abdominal muscles, excess weight, and fluid retention are all common causes. Diet and exercise can help to reduce the amount of excess weight, and help to tone the abdominal muscles. Wearing compression garments and sleeping on your left side can help to reduce fluid retention and swelling.

Will Spanx help diastasis recti?

A common post-pregnancy concern for women is diastasis recti, commonly referred to as "mommy pooch." This condition occurs when the abdominal muscles separate during pregnancy, and can often become worse after childbirth. The good news is that there are services and products available to help improve the appearance of this condition. But the question many women ask is, will Spanx help diastasis recti? Spanx is a type of shapewear that is popular among women. It is designed to smooth and slim the appearance of the body, and is often used to help improve the appearance of problem areas such as the stomach. So, it stands to reason that Spanx could help improve the appearance of diastasis recti. There is no definitive answer as to whether or not Spanx will help diastasis recti.

Every woman's body is different, and therefore every case of diastasis recti is different. Some women find that Spanx helps to improve the appearance of their diastasis recti, while others find that it does not make a noticeable difference. It is important to remember that Spanx is not a cure for diastasis recti. If you are concerned about this condition, it is best to consult with a doctor or other medical professional. They will be able to recommend the best course of treatment for you based on the severity of your case. In some cases, surgery may be the only option. If you do decide to try Spanx to help improve the appearance of diastasis recti, it is important to make sure that you are wearing the correct size. Wearing Spanx that is too small can actually make the problem worse. If you are not sure what size Spanx to buy, it is best to consult with a salesperson who can help you find the right size for your body. Spanx can be a helpful tool for some women when it comes to improving the appearance of diastasis recti. However, it is not a cure for the condition, and it is not right for everyone. If you are concerned about diastasis recti, it is best to consult with a medical professional to find out what the best course of treatment is for you.

Can you fix diastasis recti after 20 years?

It's been 20 years since you've had your baby and you're finally ready to do something about your mommy tummy. You've read all about diastasis recti and you're convinced that's what's causing your belly bulge. The big question is, can you fix diastasis recti after 20 years? Unfortunately, there is no easy answer. Diastasis recti is a separation of the abdominal muscles that can occur during pregnancy. The abdominal muscles stretch and separate to accommodate the growing baby. In most cases, the muscles will spontaneously heal after the baby is born. However, in some cases, the abdominal muscles do not completely heal, resulting in a condition called diastasis recti. There is no definitive answer as to whether or not diastasis recti can be fixed after 20 years. Some experts believe that it is possible to improve the condition with exercise and physical therapy, while others believe that it is a permanent condition. The truth is, there is no one-size-fits-all answer. Each case is unique and must be evaluated on an individual basis. If you are considering treatment for diastasis recti, it is important to consult with a qualified healthcare provider. He or she will be able to assess your individual case and determine the best course of treatment. In some cases, surgery may be necessary. However, surgery is not always successful and can often result in additional complications. Exercise and physical therapy are often recommended as a first-line treatment for diastasis recti. These treatments can help to strengthen the abdominal muscles and improve the appearance of the belly. However, it is important to note that results will vary from person to person. Some people may see a significant improvement, while others may only see a small change. If you are considering treatment for diastasis recti, it is important to set realistic expectations. There is no cure for diastasis recti and it is a condition that you will likely have to manage for the rest of your life. However, with the right treatment plan, you can improve the condition and improve your quality of life.

Do planks help diastasis recti?

When it comes to diastasis recti, or a separation of the abdominal muscles, there is a lot of debate surrounding the best course of treatment. Some people swear by planks, while others find them to be ineffective. So, what's the verdict? Can planks help diastasis recti? Separation of the abdominal muscles is a common condition, particularly among women who have been pregnant. The condition is caused by the weakening of the connective tissue that joining the right and left sides of the rectus abdominis, or the "six-pack" muscle. This can happen due to pregnancy, obesity, and even incorrect form during exercises like sit-ups and crunches. Symptoms of diastasis recti include a protruding or "pooch" belly, and discomfort or pain in the lower abdomen. The separation can also make it difficult to sit up from a lying down position, or to roll over in bed. There is no standard treatment for diastasis recti, but there are a number of exercises and therapies that can help. Planks are often recommended as a way to strengthen the abdominal muscles and help improve the condition. While there is no scientific evidence to support the claim that planks can help diastasis recti, there is some anecdotal evidence that they can be helpful. One study found that a 10-week program of therapeutic exercises, including planking, was effective in reducing the abdominal separation in women who had given birth. If you're considering trying planks to help with diastasis recti, it's important to make sure that you're doing them correctly. Incorrect form can actually make the condition worse. Always consult with a doctor or physical therapist before starting any new exercise regime. There is no one-size-fits-all solution for diastasis recti, but exercises like planks may help to improve the condition. Always consult with a doctor or physical therapist before starting any new exercise regime.

How do you know if you have Diastasis rectus abdominis?

There are several ways to determine if you have diastasis rectus abdominis (DRA). First, you can check for a separation between your abdominal muscles at the midline of your stomach. This can be done by lying on your back with your knees bent and your palms flat on the floor beside you. Next, gently press your fingertips and fingers into your stomach muscles. If you can feel a gap of more than 2.5 centimeters, you may have DRA. Another way to check for DRA is to sit up straight and place your hands on your stomach, just below your navel. As you exhale, press your stomach muscles inward. If you can feel your abdominal muscles touch, you do not have DRA. However, if you can feel a space between your muscles, you may have DRA. You may also notice that your stomach protrudes more than usual. This is because the separation between your abdominal muscles allows your intestines and other organs to push through the gap. As a result, you may notice a bulge in your stomach when you bend over or sit up. If you suspect that you have DRA, you should see a doctor for a diagnosis. DRA is often diagnosed with a physical examination and imaging tests, such as an ultrasound. Treatment for DRA typically includes exercises and physical therapy to help strengthen the muscles and help the muscles heal.

Can diastasis recti heal on its own?

The causes of diastasis recti are multi-factorial. There are many possible reasons why someone might develop this condition, including pregnancy, hormones, age, weight, and heredity. Diastasis recti refers to a separation of the rectus abdominis muscles, which are the muscles that run down the center of the stomach. This separation can cause the stomach to protrude and can lead to back pain and other issues. The good news is that diastasis recti can heal on its own. In fact, many people don't even realize they have diastasis recti until they see their doctor for another reason. If you have diastasis recti, the best thing you can do is to focus on strengthening your core muscles. This will help to close the gap between your muscles and can improve your overall health. There are a few things you can do to help diastasis recti heal on its own. First, you need to avoid any activities that put strain on your abdominals, such as sit-ups, double crunches, and leg lifts. You should also focus on strengthening your pelvic floor muscles, which can help support your abdominal muscles. Finally, you need to make sure you're getting enough rest and staying hydrated. These simple steps can go a long way in helping diastasis recti heal on its own.

What exercises should you avoid if you have diastasis recti?

If you have diastasis recti, there are certain exercises that you should avoid. These exercises can put Too much pressure on the rectus abdominis muscles and the linea alba, and can worsen the separation. Some of the exercises to avoid include: Crunches and sit-ups: These exercises can put Too much pressure on the rectus abdominis muscles and the linea alba, and can worsen the separation. Leg lifts: These exercises can also put Too much pressure on the rectus abdominis muscles and the linea alba, and can worsenthe separation. Pilates reformer exercises: Some of the exercises done on the Pilates reformer can also put Too much pressure on the rectus abdominis muscles and the linea alba, and can worsen the separation. Instead of these exercises, it is better to focus on exercises that will help to strengthen the transverse abdominis, and other core muscles. These exercises can help to take the pressure off of the rectus abdominis muscles and the linea alba, and can help to improve the separation.

This condition is often misdiagnosed as a hernia, but diastasis recti is a separation of the abdominal muscles at the midline of the body. The condition is common, affecting about one in four pregnant women and one in seven new mothers. It can also affect men, women who have never been pregnant, and people who are overweight or have chronic abdominal bloating. Diastasis recti can lead to back pain, pelvic floor dysfunction, and hernias. It can be corrected with surgery, but the best prevention is exercise during pregnancy and after childbirth.

Can you be skinny with diastasis recti?

Yes, you can be skinny with diastasis recti, but it isn't always easy. For many people, the idea of having a "perfect body" includes having toned abs. So, when you have diastasis recti (the separation of your abdominal muscles), it can be hard to feel confident about your body. Having diastasis recti doesn't mean you're overweight. In fact, people of all sizes can have this condition. The truth is, you can be skinny and have diastasis recti. There are a few things that can contribute to diastasis recti, including pregnancy, genetics, and age. If you're skinny and have diastasis recti, it may be because you've had multiple babies, you have a family history of the condition, or you're over the age of 40. So, what can you do if you're skinny and have diastasis recti? First, it's important to understand that you can't "cure" diastasis recti, but you can improve the condition. There are a number of exercises that can help to strengthen your abdominal muscles and improve the separation. If you want to try exercises at home, there are a number of online resources that can help you get started. You can also talk to your doctor or a physical therapist about exercises that may be right for you. In addition to exercise, there are other things you can do to help improve the appearance of your stomach. Wearing a supportive belly band can help to hold your muscles in place and give you the appearance of a flatter stomach. There are also a number of cosmetic procedures that can help to improve the appearance of your stomach. These include liposuction and tummy tucks. However, these procedures are typically only recommended for people who have tried exercise and other non-surgical treatments without success. If you're skinny and have diastasis recti, know that you aren't alone. There are many people in the same situation. With the right treatment and care, you can improve the appearance of your stomach and feel more confident about your body.

Who is more prone to diastasis recti?

There are a number of factors that can contribute to the development of diastasis recti. These include: - Pregnancy: The expanding belly during pregnancy puts extra pressure on the abdominal muscles, which can cause them to separate. - Weight gain: carrying extra weight, especially around the waist, can put strain on the abdominal muscles and cause them to separate. - Age: as we age, our skin and muscles lose some of their elasticity, which can make it more likely for the abdominal muscles to separate. - Genetics: some people are simply more predisposed to developing diastasis recti due to their genes. - Gender: while diastasis recti can occur in both men and women, it is more common in women. This may be due in part to the extra strain that pregnancy puts on the abdominal muscles. So, who is more prone to developing diastasis recti? Pregnancy, weight gain, age, genetics, and gender can all play a role. However, women are more likely to develop diastasis recti than men, due in part to the added strain of pregnancy on the abdominal muscles.

How much does it cost to fix diastasis recti?

According to the American Society of Plastic Surgeons, the average cost of repairing diastasis recti is $5,643. This figure will vary depending on the severity of the condition, the type of procedure performed, and the geographical location of the patient. The most common procedures used to correct diastasis recti are abdominoplasty (tummy tuck) and mini-abdominoplasty. In abdominoplasty, the surgeon will make an incision from hip to hip, and then tighten the stomach muscles and remove excess skin. In mini-abdominoplasty, the incision is smaller, and only the lower stomach muscles are tightened. The surgeon may also choose to perform liposuction to remove excess fat from the area. The cost of the procedure will also vary depending on the experience of the surgeon and the geographical location of the patient. Surgeons who perform more abdominoplasty procedures will typically charge more for their services. Patients who live in larger cities or metropolitan areas will also generally pay more for surgery due to the higher cost of living in these areas. Most insurance plans will not cover the cost of cosmetic surgery, so patients will need to pay for the procedure out of pocket. Many surgeons offer financing options to help make the procedure more affordable. Patients should consult with their surgeon to discuss all of their payment options prior to scheduling surgery.

What can worsen diastasis recti?

There are a number of things that can worsen diastasis recti. These include: - Poor posture: Slouching or slumping over can put extra pressure on your abdomen and worsen diastasis recti. - Obesity: Being overweight increases the chances of developing diastasis recti, as well as making it more difficult to recover from the condition. - Pregnancy: The added weight and pressure of pregnancy can cause or worsen diastasis recti. - Constipation: Straining to have a bowel movement can increase abdominal pressure and make diastasis recti worse. - Heavy lifting: Lifting heavy objects can also add extra pressure to your abdomen and make diastasis recti worse. If you have diastasis recti, it is important to avoid activities that may worsen your condition. If you are pregnant or overweight, you may need to seek medical help to manage your condition. Otherwise, improving your posture and avoiding heavy lifting may help to improve your symptoms.

How can I hide my diastasis recti belly?

A diastasis recti belly can be hidden by wearing clothing that is loose fitting and drapes over the stomach. This will help to camouflage the stomach and make it less noticeable. There are also some shapewear garments that can help to hold in the stomach and give the appearance of a flatter stomach. Wearing a supportive band or garment around the stomach can also help to give the appearance of a slimmer stomach.

Will planks make diastasis recti worse?

There is a lot of debate in the fitness community about whether or not planks are bad for people with diastasis recti. Some people say that planks can make the condition worse because they put extra pressure on the abdominal muscles. Others say that planks are actually helpful for people with diastasis recti because they help to strengthen the abdominal muscles. So, which is it? Can planks make diastasis recti worse? The answer is that it depends. If you have diastasis recti and you do planks without modifying them, then you could end up making your condition worse. This is because traditional planks put a lot of pressure on the abdominal muscles, which can cause the abdominal muscles to become further separated. However, if you modify your plank so that it doesn't put as much pressure on your abdominal muscles, then you can actually help to heal your diastasis recti. One way to do this is by placing a pillow or a towel under your stomach when you do a plank. This will help to take some of the pressure off of your abdominal muscles and allow them to heal. Another way to modify a plank so that it is safe for people with diastasis recti is by doing a side plank. This is a plank that is done on your side, with your weight supported by your forearm and your feet. This type of plank is much safer for people with diastasis recti because it doesn't put as much pressure on the abdominal muscles. So, if you have diastasis recti, you can still do planks. However, you need to be careful about how you do them. Make sure to modify your plank so that it is safe for you to do.

How do I close my diastasis recti gap?

A diastasis recti is a separation of the abdominal muscles that can occur during pregnancy. The gap between the muscles can vary in size, but is typically about 2.5 cm. For many women, the separation will close on its own after pregnancy. However, some women may experience a larger gap that does not close on its own. There are a few things you can do to help close the gap. First, you can try doing some exercises that target the abdominal muscles. These can include crunches, sit-ups, and plank variations. You can also focus on strengthening the muscles around the waist, such as the obliques and the lower back. Another option is to wear a support garment. This can help to hold the muscles in place and provide some compression. There are a variety of different types of support garments available, so make sure to find one that is comfortable for you to wear. If you are still pregnant, you can also try to avoid things that can contribute to the separation, such as carrying heavy objects or gaining excessive weight. After you give birth, make sure to take it easy and give your body time to recover. If you want to close your diastasis recti gap, there are a few things you can try. exercises that target the abdominal muscles, wearing a support garment, and avoiding things that can contribute to the separation.

If you have diastasis recti, you're not alone. Diastasis recti is a condition that affects many women, especially after pregnancy. Although it can be a bit uncomfortable and inconvenient, it is not a serious condition and can be treated with simple exercises and lifestyle changes. With a little patience and dedication, you can overcome this condition and get your pre-pregnancy body back!

When does diastasis need surgery?

When diastasis recti becomes severe, it may require surgery. The most common surgery for diastasis recti is called an abdominal plication. This involves sewing the separated muscles back together. This can be done through a small incision in the belly button, or through a larger incision in the lower belly. In some cases, a section of the stomach muscle may be removed. This surgery is usually done as laparoscopic surgery, which means that the surgeon makes several small incisions in the abdomen and inserts a small camera to guide the surgery.

What does a diastasis recti bulge look like?

A diastasis recti bulge may occur when the connective tissue between the right and left sides of the rectus abdominis muscle insufficiently heals following pregnancy, trauma, surgery, or aging. The resulting separation of the muscles creates a visible bulge, typically in the center of the abdomen. Although a diastasis recti bulge is usually harmless, it can cause functional and esthetic concerns. A diastasis recti bulge may be small and barely noticeable or large and visible. The size of the bulge may fluctuate depending on body position and activities. For example, the bulge may be more pronounced when lying down, coughing, or bearing down. A diastasis recti bulge may causefunctional concerns such as difficulty with bowel movements or incontinence. In some cases, the bulge may result in hernias. Esthetically, a diastasis recti bulge may be a source of body dissatisfaction. Most diastasis recti bulges do not require treatment. If treatment is desired, options include diet and exercise modifications, splinting, and surgery. Surgery is typically only recommended when other treatments have failed and the bulge is large.

What happens to your organs with diastasis recti?

With diastasis recti, the connective tissue between the left and right sides of the rectus abdominis muscle stretches. This can cause the abdominal contents to bulge outwards, and in severe cases, hernias can occur. The organs are supported by the muscular and skeletal structures of the body, and when these structures are not functioning properly, the organs can be displaced. Diastasis recti can cause the intestines and other organs to bulge out through the opening in the abdominal wall. In severe cases, hernias can occur. This can be a dangerous condition as the organs can become strangulated, or cut off from their blood supply. Diastasis recti can also cause the stomach to push up into the chest cavity (known as a hiatal hernia). This can cause heartburn, as well as difficulty swallowing and breathing. Treatment for diastasis recti often includes repairing the stretched tissue, as well as strengthening the muscles of the abdominal wall. In severe cases, surgery may be necessary to close the opening in the abdominal wall.

Are leg raises good for diastasis recti?

There is a lot of debate surrounding leg raises and whether or not they are good for diastasis recti. Those who support leg raises claim that they are an effective way to strengthen the abdominal muscles and close the gap between the abdominal muscles. However, there is no scientific evidence to support this claim. There is also a risk of further damaging the abdominal muscles or causing hernias if leg raises are not performed correctly. For people with diastasis recti, the most important thing is to focus on strengthening the abdominal muscles. This can be done through a variety of exercises, such as Pilates, yoga, and core-strengthening exercises. There is no one exercise that is guaranteed to close the gap between the abdominal muscles, but a combination of exercises that target the abdominal muscles can be effective. If you are unsure about which exercises to do, it is always a good idea to consult with a physical therapist or certified personal trainer.

Can planks fix diastasis recti?

Diastasis recti is a separation of the abdominal muscles that can occur during pregnancy. The main symptom is a protruding abdomen. Although it can be a cosmetic concern, it can also lead to Functional abdominal pain syndrome and hernias. There are a number of ways to treat diastasis recti, but one of the most popular methods is to do exercises that strengthen the abdominal muscles. One exercise that is often recommended is the plank. The plank is an excellent exercise for diastasis recti because it works all of the abdominal muscles, including the transverse abdominis, which is the muscle that helps to stabilize the spine. Planks also help to improve your posture and can help to alleviate back pain. To do a plank, you will need to get into a push-up position, but with your forearms on the ground instead of your hands. Then, you will need to hold yourself up on your toes and forearms for as long as you can. You can start by holding the position for 30 seconds and then work your way up to holding it for two minutes. If you want to see results, you need to do the plank every day. However, you should not do the plank for more than two minutes at a time because it can lead to injuries. It is also important to focus on maintaining good form throughout the exercise. When you are doing the plank, you should make sure that your back is flat, your hips are level, and your head is in line with your spine. If you start to feel pain in your back or neck, you need to stop the exercise and rest. The plank is an excellent exercise for diastasis recti, but it is not the only exercise that you can do. Other exercises that can help to strengthen the abdominal muscles include sit-ups, crunches, and squats. You can also try using a stability ball or a Pilates reformer. If you want to get rid of diastasis recti, you need to strengthen the muscles that support the spine. The best way to do this is to focus on exercises that work the whole body, including the plank.

Do all C section moms have diastasis recti?

A common concern for many women who are pregnant, or have recently given birth, is the appearance of their stomach. Stretch marks, extra skin, and a general change in shape are all normal side effects of carrying a baby. However, some women also experience a condition called diastasis recti, which can cause the stomach to protrude. So, do all c section moms have diastasis recti? The answer to this question is a bit complicated. Diastasis recti is a separation of the abdominal muscles, which can occur during pregnancy as the stomach expands. This separation can also happen during the delivery process, particularly if the baby is large or the delivery is particularly traumatic. While c section moms are more likely to experience diastasis recti, it is not a guarantee. There are a few things that c section moms can do to help prevent or reduce the severity of diastasis recti. First, it is important to maintain good posture during pregnancy and avoid activities that put unnecessary strain on the abdominal muscles, such as lifting heavy objects. Secondly, c section moms should avoid quick, jerky movements during the delivery process. And finally, c section moms should make sure to wear supportive clothing, such as a belly band, during the postpartum period to help the stomach muscles heal properly. While diastasis recti can be a concern for c section moms, it is important to remember that it is a relatively common condition and there are things that can be done to help prevent or reduce its severity.

Do you need a tummy tuck to fix diastasis recti?

A diastasis recti is a medical condition whereby the abdominal muscles separate along the midline of the stomach. This condition can cause a number of issues including back pain, hernias, and may impact the function of the abdominal muscles. A tummy tuck is a surgical procedure where the skin and fat are removed from the stomach area and the abdominal muscles are tightened. This procedure can help to alleviate the symptoms associated with a diastasis recti. It is important to note that a tummy tuck is not a cure for a diastasis recti. The abdominal muscles will still be separated, but the procedure can help to improve the appearance of the stomach and the function of the abdominal muscles. In some cases, a diastasis recti may resolve on its own without surgical intervention. However, if the separation is severe, a tummy tuck may be the best course of action. If you are considering a tummy tuck to fix a diastasis recti, it is important to consult with a board-certified plastic surgeon. The surgeon will be able to evaluate your individual case and determine whether or not a tummy tuck is right for you.

Based on the current research, it appears that diastasis recti is a relatively common condition, affecting a significant proportion of women, particularly those who are pregnant or have recently given birth. There is a lack of consensus on the best way to treat diastasis recti, but the most effective treatments appear to be exercises that focus on strengthening the deep abdominal muscles.

Can you fix diastasis recti without a tummy tuck?

Diastasis recti, or abdominal separation, is a condition that can occur during or after pregnancy. The condition is caused by the weakened and stretched abdominal muscles separating at the midline of the stomach. This can cause the stomach to protrude outward and can be painful. There are several ways to treat diastasis recti, but the most common is through surgery. Tummy tucks are the most common type of surgery to treat diastasis recti. However, there are also less invasive procedures, such as laser therapy and cortisone injections. Can you fix diastasis recti without a tummy tuck? It is possible to treat diastasis recti without surgery, but it is not always successful. nonsurgical treatments, such as physical therapy, abdominal exercises, and weight loss, can help improve the appearance of diastasis recti. However, these treatments will not work for everyone. Surgery is the most effective way to treat diastasis recti. Tummy tucks are the most common type of surgery to treat diastasis recti. Tummy tucks can remove the excess skin and fat that has stretched out the abdominal muscles. Tummy tucks can also tighten the abdominal muscles. Laser therapy is another type of surgery that can be used to treat diastasis recti. Laser therapy can help to shrink the skin and fat around the stomach. Laser therapy can also help to tighten the abdominal muscles. Cortisone injections are another type of surgery that can be used to treat diastasis recti. Cortisone injections can help to reduce the inflammation around the stomach. Cortisone injections can also help to shrink the skin and fat around the stomach. Surgery is the most effective way to treat diastasis recti. Tummy tucks are the most common type of surgery to treat diastasis recti. Tummy tucks can remove the excess skin and fat that has stretched out the abdominal muscles. Tummy tucks can also tighten the abdominal muscles. Laser therapy is another type of surgery that can be used to treat diastasis recti. Laser therapy can help to shrink the skin and fat around the stomach. Laser therapy can also help to tighten the abdominal muscles. Cortisone injections are another type of surgery that can be used to treat diastasis recti. Cortisone injections can help to reduce the inflammation around the stomach. Cortisone injections can also help to shrink the skin and fat around the stomach.

Why does diastasis recti cause a bulge?

When the abdominal muscles, specifically the rectus abdominis, separate during pregnancy, it's called diastasis recti. This separation can happen on either side of the midline or in the middle of the stomach. As the rectus abdominis muscles separate, a gap forms and the skin and intestines begin to protrude, causing a bulge. This bulge is often more noticeable when you lie down, cough, or strain. There are a few reasons why diastasis recti cause a bulge. First, the abdominal muscles are no longer supporting the spine and organs as they should. This can cause the spine to curve and the organs to sag, which can lead to a bulge. Additionally, the separation of the muscles can cause the intestines and other abdominal contents to push through the gap, leading to a bulge. Finally, pregnancy hormones can relax the connective tissue that holds the abdominal muscles in place. This can cause the muscles to separate even further and the bulge to become more pronounced. Diastasis recti is a common condition, affecting up to 60% of pregnant women. While it can be uncomfortable and cause a bulge, it is generally not harmful and will resolve on its own after pregnancy. However, there are things you can do to help manage the symptoms and reduce the risk of developing diastasis recti. Maintaining good posture, avoiding constipation, and avoiding high-impact activities can help prevent diastasis recti. If you are pregnant and experience symptoms of diastasis recti, talk to your doctor. They can provide you with advice and support to help you manage the condition.

How do you sit with diastasis recti?

How do you sit with diastasis recti? If you have diastasis recti, it's important to be mindful of how you sit. You may need to avoid sitting for long periods of time, or you may need to modify your sitting position. When sitting, be sure to: -keep your knees higher than your hips -keep your back straight -use a chair that supports your back -avoid sitting for long periods of time If you need to sit for long periods of time, be sure to take breaks often to move around and stretch. When lying down, be sure to: -place a pillow under your knees -keep your back straight -sleep on your side or on your back If you have diastasis recti, it's important to be mindful of how you sit. You may need to avoid sitting for long periods of time, or you may need to modify your sitting position. When sitting, be sure to keep your knees higher than your hips, keep your back straight, and use a chair that supports your back. Avoid sitting for long periods of time, and take breaks often to move around and stretch. When lying down, be sure to place a pillow under your knees, keep your back straight, and sleep on your side or on your back.

Can you lift weights with diastasis recti?

Whether or not you can lift weights with diastasis recti depends on the severity of your condition. If your diastasis recti is mild, you may be able to continue lifting weights without making your condition worse. However, if your diastasis recti is more severe, you may need to avoid lifting weights or only lift very light weights. If you have diastasis recti and want to start lifting weights again, it's important to consult with your doctor or physical therapist first. They can help you determine if lifting weights is safe for you and, if so, what types of exercises and weights are best. If you are cleared to lift weights, be sure to start slowly and gradually increase the amount of weight and intensity of your workouts. It's also important to focus on exercises that don't put too much strain on your abs, such as chest presses and rows. And be sure to avoid any exercises that cause pain or aggravate your symptoms. Lifting weights with diastasis recti is possible, but it's important to be cautious and consult with a medical professional before starting any new exercise routine.

What is the best exercise for separated stomach muscles?

Out of all the exercises that help with diastasis recti, the best one is the Pilates reformer. This machine uses springs and pulleys to provide resistance as you move, making it ideal for toning your deep abdominal muscles. The resistance offered by the reformer also helps to close the gap between your separated stomach muscles.

Can a chiropractor fix diastasis recti?

Diastasis recti is a condition that can occur during or after pregnancy, and it refers to the separation of the rectus abdominis muscles. This can cause the stomach to protrude and can be painful. Some women may also experience back pain and incontinence. Chiropractors are often sought out for help with diastasis recti, as they are trained in manipulating the spine and other joints. There is no evidence that chiropractic care can directly fix diastasis recti, but it may help to ease some of the symptoms associated with it. In particular, chiropractic care may help to relieve back pain and improve incontinence. If you are considering seeing a chiropractor for diastasis recti, it is important to find one who is experienced in treating this condition.

Which hormones causes rectus abdominis diastasis?

Hormones are important regulators of many bodily functions, and they can also play a role in the development of certain conditions. In the case of rectus abdominis diastasis, there are a few hormones that may be involved in the condition. One hormone that has been studied in relation to rectus abdominis diastasis is relaxin. Relaxin is a hormone that is produced by the body during pregnancy, and it helps to loosen the joints and ligaments in preparation for childbirth. It is thought that relaxin may also play a role in the development of rectus abdominis diastasis, as it can weaken the connective tissue that holds the abdominal muscles together. Another hormone that has been studied in relation to rectus abdominis diastasis is estrogen. Estrogen is a hormone that is produced by the ovaries, and it is involved in the development of female sexual characteristics. Estrogen levels vary throughout the menstrual cycle, and they can also fluctuate during pregnancy. Some research has suggested that high levels of estrogen may contribute to the development of rectus abdominis diastasis. Progesterone is another hormone that has been studied in relation to rectus abdominis diastasis. Progesterone is a hormone that is produced by the ovaries, and it is involved in the development of the lining of the uterus. Progesterone levels also fluctuate throughout the menstrual cycle and during pregnancy. Some research has suggested that high levels of progesterone may contribute to the development of rectus abdominis diastasis. These are just a few of the hormones that have been studied in relation to rectus abdominis diastasis. It is possible that other hormones may also play a role in the condition. However, more research is needed to better understand the role of hormones in the development of rectus abdominis diastasis.

A diastasis recti is a separation of the abdominal muscles that can occur during pregnancy. This can lead to back pain and other issues. While there is no cure, there are treatments that can help to improve the condition.

How can you tell the difference between diastasis recti and fat?

There are a few key ways to tell the difference between diastasis recti and fat. First, diastasis recti will often present as a protrusion or bulge in the stomach area, while fat is more likely to be distributed evenly throughout the body. Second, diastasis recti will typically affect both the rectus abdominis ("six pack") muscles and theexternal obliques (side waist muscles), while fat is more likely to only impact the rectus abdominis. Finally, diastasis recti may be accompanied by other symptoms like back pain or difficulty breathing, while fat typically will not. Of course, the best way to definitively tell the difference between diastasis recti and fat is to consult with a doctor or other medical professional. They will be able to perform a physical examination and may order additional tests like an ultrasound or MRI to get a better look at the tissues in question.

Can diastasis recti close on its own?

There is no right or wrong answer to this question. Each individual case is unique and will require different care. Speak with your doctor to determine the best course of action for you. In general, diastasis recti—or abdominal separation—is a condition that can affect both men and women, though it is most common among pregnant women and new moms. The condition occurs when the rectus abdominis muscles, which run down the center of the stomach from the rib cage to the pelvis, separate at the midline. This can happen due to pregnancy, obesity, or genetics. While diastasis recti can cause some cosmetic concerns, it is generally not a harmful condition. However, it can lead to back pain and weak abdominal muscles. In severe cases, hernias can develop. Most cases of diastasis recti can be improved with lifestyle changes, such as exercise and weight loss. For some women, surgery may be necessary to repair the abdominal muscles. So, can diastasis recti close on its own? In some cases, yes. However, it is important to speak with your doctor to determine the best course of action for you.

How long does it take to close diastasis recti with exercise?

How long does it take to close diastasis recti with exercise? The time required to close diastasis recti through exercise will vary depending on the individual. For some, it may only take a few weeks or months to see results. However, for others, it may take longer. The severity of the condition will also play a role in how long it will take to improve. Those with a more severe case of diastasis recti may need to put in more time and effort to close the gap. Regardless of the individual case, it is important to be patient and consistent with the exercises. Closure of diastasis recti is possible with exercise and patience.

Are standing ABS good for diastasis recti?

There is a lot of debate surrounding whether or not standing abs are good for diastasis recti. Some people argue that they are helpful because they help to engage the transverse abdominis, which can help to close the gap between the abdominal muscles. Others argue that standing abs can actually make the separation worse because they put unnecessary pressure on the abdominal muscles. There is no right or wrong answer, and ultimately it is up to the person with diastasis recti to decide what exercises are best for them. If someone is experiencing a lot of pain or discomfort when doing standing abs, it may be best to avoid them. However, if someone finds that they are able to do them without pain, then they may be a helpful exercise to do.

How do you tighten abs with diastasis recti?

There are a number of ways you can go about tightening your abs when you have diastasis recti. One option is to do specific exercises that help to target the area. This might involve things like planks, sit-ups, and other core strengthening exercises. You can also try wearing a compression garment, which can help to hold everything in place and give you the feeling of having a tighter stomach. Additionally, you can work on your posture and make sure you're not putting any extra strain on your midsection. By doing all of these things, you can help to improve the appearance of your stomach and make your abs look tighter.

What exercises heal diastasis recti?

A recent study published in the journal Physical Therapy found that exercises that place a focus on strengthening the transverse abdominal muscles may help to improve symptoms associated with diastasis recti. The condition, which is more commonly seen in pregnant women, is characterized by a separation of the rectus abdominis muscles. This can often lead to a bulge in the abdomen and/or lower back pain. The study authors note that while there is no "cure" for diastasis recti, treatments that focus on strengthening the transverse abdominis muscle may help to improve symptoms and quality of life for those affected. They add that the exercises included in their study were found to be safe and effective in a small group of participants, and may offer a "conservative and feasible" option for the treatment of diastasis recti. So, what exercises can you do to help heal diastasis recti? The following exercises are a great place to start: Pelvic Tilts: This is a great exercise to help strengthen the lower abdominals and improve your posture. To perform a pelvic tilt, start by lying on your back with your knees bent and feet flat on the ground. Slowly arch your back, pressing your pelvis towards the ceiling. Hold for a count of five, then return to the starting position. Repeat 10 times. Crunches: This classic exercise is a great way to target the rectus abdominis muscle. To perform a crunch, lie on your back with your knees bent and feet flat on the floor. Place your hands behind your head and gently pull your head and shoulders off the ground. Hold for a count of five, then slowly return to the starting position. Repeat 10 times. Bicycle Crunches: This variation of the classic crunch targets the obliques, which are the muscles that run along the sides of your waist. To perform bicycle crunches, lie on your back with your knees bent and feet flat on the floor. Place your hands behind your head and gently pull your head and shoulders off the ground. As you lift your shoulders, bring your right knee in towards your chest while extending your left leg out straight. Hold for a count of five, then switch sides and repeat. Continue alternating sides for a total of 10 repetitions. Planks: This is a great exercise for the entire core, including the transverse abdominis muscle. To perform a plank, start by lying on your stomach with your elbows bent and palms flat on the ground. Push up onto your forearms and toes, keeping your body in a straight line from your head to your heels. Hold for a count of 10, then lower back down to the starting position. Repeat 10 times. While there is no "cure" for diastasis recti, the good news is that there are exercises that can help to improve symptoms and quality of life for those affected

Diastasis recti is an abdominal condition that occurs when the abdominal muscles separate. This condition is common in pregnant women and can also be seen in men and women who are overweight. Although diastasis recti is not a dangerous condition, it can lead to hernias and other abdominal problems. Treatment for diastasis recti includes core strengthening exercises and weight loss. Surgery is rarely necessary.

SD - #0052 - 140926 - C0 - 229/152/9 - PB - 9781776969807 - Matt Lamination